The Power of Cellular Health

Secrets to a Longer, Happier Life

By:

Margaret Price

TABLE OF CONTENTS

INTRODUCTION

Unlocking the Secrets of Cellular Health for Longevity and Happiness

Understanding Cellular Health: Why It Matters More Than Ever

The Science of Aging and Cellular Vitality

How to Use This Book for Lasting Change and Immediate Results

CHAPTER 1: The Foundation of Vitality – Understanding Cellular Energy

The Role of Mitochondria as Your Body's Powerhouse

How to Spot Early Signs of Cellular Decline

Building Cellular Resilience Through Simple Daily Habits

A Look at the Potential Long-Term Benefits

Practical Tips to Start Today

Embracing a Cellular Mindset for Lasting Change

CHAPTER 2: Embracing Gut Health as the Gateway to Longevity

Why Gut Health is Crucial for Cellular Longevity

The Gut-Cellular Health Connection in Action

Top Nutritional Strategies for a Healthy Gut

Addressing Inflammation: The Root of Cellular Aging

Foods and Habits to Reduce Gut-Related Inflammation

Putting It All Together: A Holistic Approach to Gut and Cellular Health

CHAPTER 3: The Power of Cellular Detox – Cleansing for Optimal Function

Identifying and Eliminating Toxins from Your Environment

Practical Steps for Daily Detoxification

Natural Supplements and Herbs to Support Cellular Detox

CHAPTER 4: Reclaiming Energy – From Fatigue to Vitality

Key Causes of Low Energy and How to Address Them

Simple Lifestyle Changes to Boost Cellular Energy

Nourishing Your Cells for Sustainable Energy All Day

CHAPTER 5: The Essential Role of Sunlight in Cellular Health

How Sunlight Impacts Your Cellular and Mitochondrial Health

Optimizing Vitamin D and Circadian Rhythms Naturally

1. The Importance of Vitamin D for Cellular Health

Strategies to Safely Incorporate Sun Exposure in Daily Life

Embracing the Healing Power of Sunlight

CHAPTER 6: Movement and Exercise for Cell Renewal and Longevity

The Science Behind Exercise and Cellular Rejuvenation

Tailored Exercise Plans for All Fitness Levels

How to Incorporate Movement into a Busy Lifestyle

Embrace Movement as Part of Your Cellular Health Journey

CHAPTER 7: Cellular Nutrition – Eating to Fuel Longevity

Embracing Healthy Fats, Carbs, and Proteins for Cellular Health

The Impact of Sugar, Processed Foods, and Inflammation on Cells

Easy-to-Follow Meal Plans for Optimal Cell Function

Tips for Making the Meal Plan Work for You

Embracing Cellular Nutrition for Long-Term Health

CHAPTER 8: Healthy Fats and Oils – Rejuvenating Your Cells

Understanding the Importance of Healthy Fats

Why Fat Quality Matters

Common Cooking Oils to Avoid and What to Use Instead

CHAPTER 9: Collagen and Protein – Building Blocks for Cellular Repair

The Role of Collagen in Cellular Health and Anti-Aging

How Collagen Supports Anti-Aging and Cellular Repair

How to Incorporate Collagen into Your Diet

How to Choose the Right Protein Sources for Longevity

Daily Strategies to Support Protein Synthesis and Cell Repair

Embracing the Power of Protein and Collagen for Cellular Health

CHAPTER 10: Gut Repair and Immune Strengthening Through Smart Carbs

How Carbohydrates Support Gut and Cellular Health

Choosing the Right Carbs for Optimal Immune Support

Sample Recipes to Fuel Gut Repair and Cellular Vitality

Daily Strategies to Support Protein Synthesis and Cell Repair

Final Thoughts on Gut Repair and Immune Strengthening

CHAPTER 11: Cellular-Boosting Supplements for Mitochondrial Health

An Overview of Essential Vitamins and Supplements

Safe Usage and Potential Side Effects to Be Aware Of

Building a Supplement Routine for Daily Energy and Health

Empowering Your Cells for a Life of Vitality

CHAPTER 12: Empowering Your Metabolism – The 30-Day Cellular Health Plan

A Step-by-Step Plan to Jumpstart Your Cellular Renewal

Daily Practices to Boost Energy, Mood, and Vitality

Tracking Progress and Celebrating Your Health Journey

Chapter 13: Thriving in a Modern World – Sustaining Cellular Health

Addressing Modern Stressors That Impact Cellular Well-Being

Tools and Resources for Continued Cellular Health Success

Embracing Cellular Health for Life

CONCLUSION: Embracing the Power of Cellular Health for a Life of Vitality and Joy

Honoring Your Body's Potential

A Lifelong Commitment to Wellness

Share Your Journey with Others

INTRODUCTION

Unlocking the Secrets of Cellular Health for Longevity and Happiness

Imagine waking up each morning filled with energy and focus, ready to take on the day with a deep sense of vitality. Imagine consistently feeling that way regardless of age or life's demands.

Many of us have dreamt of this energy, only to be met by persistent fatigue, fogginess, or other signs of aging that seem unavoidable. But what if these weren't just symptoms of "getting older" but signs that your cells—your body's fundamental building blocks—are calling for more care?

My own journey began during a period of unrelenting exhaustion and physical weariness. I was juggling a career, family responsibilities, and personal aspirations, but I felt as if my body was resisting me at every step.

No matter how much rest I got or how carefully I watched my diet, my energy lagged, my mind felt foggy, and my mood was erratic.

Traditional advice only helped temporarily, and I knew I needed a more profound solution.

My search led me to discover the concept of cellular health. Through my mentors—world-renowned experts like Dr. Megan Rossi, Rhiannon Lambert, and Dr. Philip Goglia—I learned that optimal health isn't just about managing symptoms; it's about nurturing the cells that make us who we are.

In time, I understood that actual vitality begins at the cellular level. When our cells thrive, we feel energized, resilient, and alive. The Power of Cellular Health is the culmination of that journey, and it's my guide for you to experience the transformative power of nurturing your cells.

Understanding Cellular Health: Why It Matters More Than Ever

In today's world, our cells face unprecedented challenges. Every day, they're bombarded by stress, environmental toxins, poor diet, lack of sleep, and a fast-paced lifestyle that takes a toll over time. These stressors chip away at our health, slowly depleting the very foundation of our vitality.

The problem is that traditional health solutions often address the symptoms—fatigue, sluggishness, or irritability—rather than the root causes. It's like putting a bandage over a wound without treating the underlying infection. So, we keep going, wondering why our energy dips in the afternoon or why we can't concentrate for more than a few minutes.

That's where cellular health comes in. This book will guide you to understand how to protect, rejuvenate, and nourish your cells so they can perform their best. Each cell is like a small engine in your body, powering everything you do, from thinking clearly to staying active.

Caring for our cells addresses health at its root, creating a solid foundation supporting every aspect of our well-being. When prioritizing cellular health, we create a ripple effect that improves our energy, mood, mental clarity, and resilience.

One of the critical discoveries in cellular health is that there is always time to start making improvements. Small changes can lead to significant, lasting benefits regardless of age or current health. You can reverse some of the wear and tear through simple, science-backed practices, helping your cells regenerate, repair, and function as designed. Cellular health doesn't just help you live longer; it helps you live better.

The Science of Aging and Cellular Vitality

Aging is a natural process, but how we age is largely up to us. Every year, our cells experience wear and tear as they perform the thousands of functions necessary for survival. Our cells repair, divide, and adapt to keep us healthy, but this maintenance becomes more challenging over time. Cellular damage accumulates, and our cells struggle with the tasks they once managed easily.

Research reveals that aging is not merely a decline; it's a gradual change at the cellular level that we can influence. By addressing cellular health, we give our cells the support they need to maintain vitality as we age.

This is where mitochondria, our cells' energy generators, play a crucial role. Mitochondria take the oxygen and food we breathe and transform them into energy. As we age, mitochondria become less efficient, leading to fatigue, decreased mental clarity, and weakened resilience.

But here's the good news: mitochondrial function can be supported and improved. Through targeted nutrition, lifestyle adjustments, and supplements, we can enhance mitochondrial health and, in turn, boost our energy and vitality. This book will take you through the key strategies for supporting mitochondrial function, from dietary adjustments to specific exercises and stress management techniques.

Beyond mitochondria, cellular health involves understanding the gut microbiome, a crucial network of bacteria in our intestines. These bacteria interact with our cells to support immune function, nutrient absorption, and mental health. A healthy gut microbiome is a foundation for overall cellular health, allowing nutrients to reach our cells and toxins to be effectively eliminated.

The science of aging and cellular health may sound complex. Still, the principles are straightforward: by providing our cells with the nutrients, rest, and care they need, we empower them to perform at their best, creating a body that ages with strength and resilience rather than decline.

How to Use This Book for Lasting Change and Immediate Results

The Power of Cellular Health is not about quick fixes or fleeting health trends. Instead, it's a roadmap to building a lifestyle that honors your cells and unlocks your vitality. This book combines the latest scientific insights with actionable, practical steps to experience a transformation beyond temporary relief.

Here's how to use it:

- Start with the Basics: The early chapters lay the foundation of cellular health. By understanding how cells function and what they need to thrive, you'll be prepared to make meaningful changes in your life.

- Implement the Action Steps Gradually: Each chapter concludes with practical advice you can implement immediately. You don't need to overhaul your life overnight; instead, try incorporating one or two changes at a time.

Gradual progress leads to lasting habits, and you'll likely notice minor improvements that motivate you to continue.

- Customize Your Journey: Cellular health is adaptable. Only some strategies will work perfectly for everyone, so this book offers a variety of options. Choose what aligns with your lifestyle and needs, whether it's nutritional shifts, exercise routines, or stress management techniques.

- Track Your Transformation: Pay attention to the changes you feel as you integrate cellular health into your life. Notice how your energy levels improve, your focus sharpens, and your mood stabilizes. These changes are signs that your cells are responding, motivating them to continue.

- Keep Learning and Adapting: Cellular health is an evolving field. While this book provides a comprehensive guide, new research and discoveries will always occur. Think of this as the beginning of a journey that invites you to keep exploring and adapting for long-term wellness.

As you begin this journey into cellular health, remember that every step you take is an investment in a life of vibrancy and resilience. Whether seeking more energy, greater clarity, or a sense of well-being, nurturing your cells is the key to unlocking these gifts. The potential to thrive, no matter your age, is within you, and this book will empower you to achieve it.

In the following chapters, you'll discover that cellular health isn't about reaching a perfect state but about learning to support and appreciate your body at every age. Through this journey, you're not just adding years to your life—you're adding life to your years. So, let's dive in and explore the power of cellular health together, one step at a time. Your body, mind, and future self will thank you.

CHAPTER 1: The Foundation of Vitality – Understanding Cellular Energy

In our fast-paced world, energy is one of our most precious resources. It's what powers us to work, to connect with others, and to pursue our goals and passions. Yet, for many, that energy seems elusive.

You're not alone if you've ever felt persistently tired, struggling to stay focused, or constantly battling fatigue. Traditional approaches often attribute these feelings to stress, poor sleep, or simply getting older. But the root of these symptoms goes deeper—to the very cells that power our bodies.

Welcome to the foundation of vitality: cellular energy. Understanding how your cells produce and sustain energy is vital to feeling vibrant and energized.

This chapter will explore the role of mitochondria, often called the "powerhouses" of our cells, how to recognize early signs of cellular decline, and simple yet powerful habits to keep your cells—and you—operating at their best.

The Role of Mitochondria as Your Body's Powerhouse

Mitochondria are tiny structures within your cells responsible for producing the energy you use for everything you do. They take the oxygen and food you breathe and convert them into ATP (adenosine triphosphate), which powers nearly every cellular function. Without healthy mitochondria, you'd be unable to move, think, or even breathe.

When our mitochondria function well, they supply energy efficiently, keeping us active and alert. However, over time, mitochondria face various stressors—like poor diet, environmental toxins, and chronic stress—that compromise their efficiency. This process, known as mitochondrial dysfunction, is often at the core of persistent fatigue, reduced cognitive function, and other health issues.

For example, let's consider fatigue. Imagine your mitochondria as the battery in your phone. When fully charged and functioning well, the phone can last all day. But if the battery starts to wear out, it only holds a charge for as long as possible, and you find yourself reaching for the charger more frequently. Similarly, when your mitochondria are damaged or depleted, your cells can't produce as much energy, leaving you feeling drained and sluggish even after a whole night's rest.

Many people in today's world are experiencing mitochondrial dysfunction without even knowing it. This process happens gradually, often going unnoticed until symptoms become too difficult to ignore. Fortunately, by supporting mitochondrial health, you can improve energy levels, boost mental clarity, and even slow down the effects of aging.

How to Spot Early Signs of Cellular Decline

Recognizing the signs of cellular and mitochondrial decline early on is crucial to taking action before more serious health issues arise. When our mitochondria struggle, our entire body feels the effects, but these signs are often subtle initially.

1. Persistent Fatigue

One of the most common signs of cellular decline is unrelenting fatigue that doesn't go away with rest. If you need multiple cups of coffee to make it through the day or wake up tired even after a whole night's sleep, your mitochondria may struggle to meet your energy demands.

2. Brain Fog and Reduced Mental Clarity

Mitochondria are responsible for physical energy and play a vital role in brain health. When they're underperforming, it can lead to cognitive symptoms like brain fog, difficulty concentrating, and memory lapses.

For example, have you ever walked into a room and forgotten why or struggled to remember a simple detail you knew moments before? These can be signs that your brain cells aren't getting the energy they need.

3. Slow Recovery from Physical Activity

If it takes you longer to recover from physical exertion than it used to, mitochondrial decline may be at play. Mitochondria are particularly important in muscle cells, which rely heavily on ATP during physical activity. When mitochondria are compromised, your muscles have more difficulty repairing and recovering, leading to prolonged soreness and fatigue after exercise.

4. Aging Skin and Visible Signs of Aging

Mitochondria also contribute to skin health by supporting cell renewal and repair. When they're functioning well, your skin appears vibrant and resilient. But when mitochondrial function declines, it can lead to dull skin, fine lines, and other visible signs of aging.

These early indicators of cellular decline signal that your body needs support. By recognizing these signs, you can act before they become more severe health issues.

Building Cellular Resilience Through Simple Daily Habits

The good news is that supporting mitochondrial health doesn't require drastic changes. Small, consistent habits can go a long way in protecting and rejuvenating your mitochondria, helping you regain energy and vitality over time.

Here are some of the most effective habits you can adopt:

1. Prioritize Nutrient-Dense Foods

Mitochondria rely on specific nutrients to function optimally, including B vitamins, magnesium, CoQ10, and omega-3 fatty acids. A diet rich in colorful fruits, vegetables, lean proteins, and healthy fats provides these essential nutrients and supports mitochondrial function.

For example, leafy greens like spinach and kale are high in B vitamins, which are crucial for energy production. Fatty fish, like salmon, provide omega-3s that support mitochondrial membranes, helping them maintain structural integrity.

Avoid processed foods and excess sugars, which create oxidative stress and inflammation, both harmful to mitochondria. Think of it as choosing fuel for your body: whole foods provide clean energy, while processed foods bog down your system and reduce efficiency.

2. Incorporate Movement into Your Day

Regular exercise is one of the most powerful tools for enhancing mitochondrial health. Physical activity stimulates mitochondria to produce more ATP and even prompts your body to create new mitochondria, especially in muscle cells. Start with activities you enjoy— walking, swimming, yoga, or weightlifting—and aim to move daily. High-intensity interval training (HIIT) efficiently boosts mitochondrial function, as it challenges your muscles in a way that encourages mitochondrial adaptation.

Even if you're busy, simple actions like taking the stairs, going for short walks throughout the day, or stretching at your desk can make a difference.

3. Get Quality Sleep

During sleep, your body repairs and rejuvenates itself, which includes cellular maintenance. Poor sleep harms mitochondrial function, disrupting the body's ability to produce ATP efficiently.

To improve sleep quality, create a bedtime routine that encourages relaxation, limit exposure to screens in the hour before bed, and aim for 7-8 hours of uninterrupted sleep each night.

Think of sleep as an essential recharge for your cells. Just as you wouldn't expect your phone to function well without charging, your body needs sleep to keep your cells running optimally.

4. Reduce Toxin Exposure and Practice Regular Detoxification

Environmental toxins, such as pollution, chemicals in household products, and pesticides in food, can damage mitochondria over time. While avoiding all toxins is impossible, you can reduce your exposure by choosing organic foods when possible, using natural cleaning products, and avoiding plastics that contain harmful chemicals like BPA.

Additionally, consider practices that support your body's natural detoxification processes, such as drinking plenty of water, eating fiber-rich foods, and incorporating antioxidant-rich foods like berries. These small steps help your body eliminate toxins more effectively, easing the burden on your mitochondria.

5. Manage Stress Effectively

Chronic stress releases cortisol, a hormone that can damage mitochondria when elevated for extended periods. Practicing stress management techniques, such as deep breathing, mindfulness, or spending time in nature, can help keep cortisol levels in check. Regularly setting aside time for relaxation is good for your mind and essential for cellular health.

For example, try a simple breathing exercise: inhale for a count of four, hold for four, exhale for four, and hold for four. Repeat this daily for a few minutes to reduce stress and support your cellular health.

6. Embrace the Power of Sunlight

Sunlight is not only uplifting but also essential for cellular health. Exposure to natural light, especially in the morning, helps regulate your body's circadian rhythm, supporting mitochondrial function and overall energy levels. Sunlight enables your body to produce vitamin D, crucial in immune health and cellular repair.

Aim to spend at least 10–20 minutes outside each morning, even if it's overcast. By exposing your skin and eyes to natural light, you're boosting vitamin D levels and signaling to your mitochondria that it's time to be active and energized. Try pairing this with a gentle morning walk or stretching session for a double benefit—movement and sunlight working together to kickstart your day.

7. Incorporate Breathing Exercises and Oxygenate Your Cells

Oxygen is essential for cellular energy production, as it's a core component in ATP synthesis within your mitochondria. While we naturally breathe all day, most take shallow breaths, limiting the oxygen available to our cells. Deep breathing exercises can increase oxygen flow, boosting your cells and enhancing mitochondrial efficiency.

A simple technique is diaphragmatic breathing, where you focus on breathing deeply into your belly instead of just your chest. Inhale slowly for a count of four, letting your stomach expand, hold for four, then exhale for four, fully emptying your lungs.

Repeat for a few minutes each day. Over time, this practice can improve cellular oxygenation, reduce stress, and improve overall energy levels.

8. Stay Hydrated to Support Cellular Efficiency

Water is the primary medium for all cellular functions, including energy production. When you're dehydrated, cellular processes slow down, and mitochondria struggle to produce ATP efficiently. Dehydration also contributes to fatigue, brain fog, and reduced endurance—symptoms often attributed to other causes.

Make it a habit to drink water consistently throughout the day. Adding a pinch of sea salt or a slice of lemon can help enhance electrolyte balance, which supports cellular function.

Aim for around half of your body weight in ounces of water daily (e.g., if you weigh 150 pounds, drink about 75 ounces). Staying hydrated might seem simple, but it can profoundly impact your energy levels and cellular health.

A Look at the Potential Long-Term Benefits

Supporting your mitochondria and building cellular resilience through daily habits doesn't just impact how you feel today—it can profoundly affect your long-term health. Studies suggest that mitochondrial health is linked to everything from cognitive longevity to reduced risk of chronic diseases, such as heart disease, diabetes, and neurodegenerative conditions.

Consider brain health as an example. Research has shown that mitochondrial dysfunction in the brain cells is associated with cognitive decline and conditions like Alzheimer's.

By supporting mitochondrial function through proper nutrition, movement, and stress management, you can maintain cognitive clarity and protect against future cognitive impairment. Think of it as a long-term investment in your mental sharpness and memory retention.

Similarly, mitochondrial health plays a role in preventing inflammation—a key driver of many age-related diseases. Inflammation often begins at the cellular level, and when mitochondria are damaged, they release inflammatory signals. By supporting mitochondria, you're helping reduce chronic inflammation, supporting a healthier immune response, and decreasing the risk of inflammatory diseases.

Practical Tips to Start Today

You can implement only some strategies at a time. Start with a few manageable changes, such as adding more nutrient-dense foods, committing to regular movement, or focusing on your sleep routine. As you start noticing improvements, it will motivate you to continue building on these habits.

For example, you might begin by improving your diet with one new habit each week. Start by incorporating more leafy greens, rich in B vitamins and magnesium—essential for mitochondrial function. Next week, add a serving of fatty fish like salmon, which is rich in omega-3 fatty acids that help protect cell membranes. You'll have created a dietary foundation that significantly supports cellular energy in a month.

Similarly, if exercise feels overwhelming, start small with just a 10-minute daily walk. Gradually increase this time and incorporate different forms of movement, like strength training or yoga, which enhance cellular function and support mental well-being.

Embracing a Cellular Mindset for Lasting Change

While some health trends promise quick results, cellular health is a lifelong commitment to wellness. As you adopt these practices, you're creating a ripple effect throughout your body that builds a foundation of resilience and strength. You're no longer just focusing on fixing symptoms but are supporting the very source of your energy and vitality.

Adopting a "cellular mindset" means viewing each choice as a way to nurture and protect your cells. The food you eat, how you manage stress, the time you spend in the sun, and the rest you prioritize all contribute to a healthier, more resilient body.

This mindset shift moves you away from a reactive approach to health and toward a proactive, sustainable model that empowers you to feel your best, year after year.

Moving Forward

Throughout the rest of this book, we'll explore specific topics to support your journey. You'll learn how to use nutrients, supplements, detox practices, and more to create a cellular environment that promotes optimal health. Each chapter builds on the previous one, helping you deepen your understanding and giving you actionable steps to create a life of energy and well-being.

As you move forward, remember that small steps add up. Building cellular resilience doesn't require perfection—it's about progress. Every positive choice you make today invests in a brighter, healthier tomorrow. Embrace the journey, celebrate your progress, and know that you're unlocking the potential for a vibrant, fulfilling life by supporting your cells.

CHAPTER 2: Embracing Gut Health as the Gateway to Longevity

In the journey toward cellular health and longevity, it's easy to overlook one of the most critical contributors to well-being: the gut. Known as the "second brain," our gut influences every aspect of our health, from immune function to mood regulation, and is intricately tied to how our cells perform, age, and regenerate.

Recent research has revealed that a thriving gut microbiome—the diverse community of bacteria and microorganisms in our digestive tract—is essential to unlocking vitality and longevity.

This chapter will explore the powerful connection between your gut microbiome and cellular health, the most effective nutritional strategies for promoting a healthy gut, and how managing inflammation can significantly slow cellular aging.

By the end, you will understand how gut health is the foundation of lasting vitality, clear energy, and true wellness.

Why Gut Health is Crucial for Cellular Longevity

The cells in your body work tirelessly to keep you functioning, but for them to perform optimally, they need a healthy environment and the proper nutrients.

This is where the gut microbiome comes in; comprising trillions of bacteria, fungi, and other microorganisms, the gut microbiome plays a central role in nutrient absorption, immune defense, and waste elimination, which are crucial for cellular health.

A balanced gut microbiome aids in breaking down complex carbohydrates, producing essential nutrients like B vitamins and vitamin K, and generating short-chain fatty acids that provide energy and regulate immune function. When our gut is thriving, our cells receive a steady supply of nutrients and protection, which enables them to carry out vital processes efficiently.

On the flip side, an imbalanced gut microbiome lacking diversity or dominated by harmful bacteria can disrupt nutrient absorption, weaken immunity, and lead to chronic inflammation. Over time, these effects take a toll on our cells, accelerating cellular aging and contributing to fatigue, cognitive decline, and vulnerability to illness. Cultivating a healthy gut microbiome is crucial in establishing the cellular foundation for a longer, more resilient life.

The Gut-Cellular Health Connection in Action

To illustrate the importance of this connection, consider a common scenario: a person experiencing ongoing digestive issues, fatigue, and mood swings. These symptoms are often linked to an unhealthy gut, which impairs the absorption of essential nutrients like magnesium, omega-3 fatty acids, and vitamin D—nutrients essential for energy production, immune function, and brain health.

Without an adequate nutrient supply, the mitochondria (the energy-producing structures within cells) can't perform efficiently, leading to low energy, weakened immunity, and mental fog. This example highlights gut health, which supports cellular function, energy, and resilience.

Top Nutritional Strategies for a Healthy Gut

Nurturing your gut microbiome doesn't have to be complicated. Focusing on critical nutritional strategies allows you to build a balanced and diverse gut environment that supports your cells from within. These strategies are sustainable, evidence-based, and easy to incorporate daily.

1. Prioritize Prebiotic-Rich Foods

Prebiotics are non-digestible fibers that feed beneficial bacteria in your gut. By feeding these "good" bacteria, prebiotics promote a balanced microbiome, helping healthy microbes flourish and preventing harmful bacteria from taking over.

Including prebiotics in your diet supports digestion, enhances immune response, and improves nutrient absorption, which is vital for cellular health.

Examples of Prebiotic-Rich Foods:

- Garlic: Rich in inulin, garlic promotes beneficial bacteria growth and reduces inflammation.

- Onions: They contain prebiotic fibers that boost gut health and are also high in antioxidants.

- Leeks: High in fiber and prebiotics, leeks support the gut and add flavor to meals.

- Bananas: Green bananas, notably, contain resistant starch, a type of prebiotic fiber that supports gut health and balances blood sugar.

Tip: Add garlic and onions to your meals as natural flavor boosters, or enjoy a banana as a snack. Simple, consistent additions like these can profoundly affect your gut microbiome.

2. Incorporate Probiotic-Rich Foods

Probiotics are live beneficial bacteria that can restore and maintain gut balance. Various probiotic-rich foods can enhance digestion, increase immune resilience, and improve mental clarity by supporting nutrient absorption and healthy gut-brain communication.

Examples of Probiotic Foods:

- Yogurt: Choose plain, unsweetened yogurt with live cultures to avoid added sugars.

- Kimchi: This Korean dish is packed with probiotics and rich in vitamins.

- Sauerkraut: Fermented cabbage that's high in probiotics, perfect for salads or as a side.

- Kefir: A fermented milk drink similar to yogurt but with a broader range of beneficial bacteria.

Tip: Add a small serving of fermented foods to your meals a few times weekly. The beneficial bacteria introduced through probiotics can help diversify your gut microbiome and support nutrient absorption.

3. Eat High-Fiber Foods for Optimal Digestion

Fiber is essential for maintaining a balanced gut. It promotes regularity, supports blood sugar stability, and serves as fuel for gut bacteria. Fiber also helps build a strong gut barrier, preventing harmful substances from leaking into the bloodstream and triggering inflammation.

Examples of High-Fiber Foods:

- Chia Seeds: High in fiber and omega-3s, chia seeds support gut health and reduce inflammation.

- Oats: Rich in beta-glucan, a soluble fiber that nourishes gut bacteria.

- Beans and Lentils: These legumes are excellent sources of fiber, promoting fullness and supporting digestion.

Tip: Add chia seeds to your breakfast or snack on fiber-rich vegetables and fruits throughout the day. These small, consistent choices support a balanced microbiome, improving digestion and nutrient absorption.

Addressing Inflammation: The Root of Cellular Aging

One of the most profound benefits of supporting your gut microbiome is its role in reducing inflammation, a major contributor to cellular aging. Inflammation is a natural defense mechanism, but chronic inflammation—often driven by poor diet, stress, and a lack of microbial diversity—takes a toll on the body over time. Left unchecked, it can accelerate cellular damage, reducing the efficiency of cellular repair and regeneration.

An unbalanced gut microbiome can contribute to chronic inflammation through a condition known as "leaky gut."

When the gut lining is compromised, harmful substances such as undigested food particles and toxins can leak into the bloodstream, triggering an immune response and increasing inflammation. Over time, this can strain the immune system, weaken cellular function, and hasten aging.

Foods and Habits to Reduce Gut-Related Inflammation

By making intentional dietary changes and incorporating specific habits, you can reduce inflammation and protect your cells from accelerated aging.

1. Minimize Refined Sugar and Processed Foods

Processed foods and refined sugars feed harmful bacteria and contribute to inflammation in the gut. Reducing your intake of sugary snacks, refined grains, and artificial additives can help restore gut balance and reduce inflammatory responses.

2. Embrace Anti-Inflammatory Foods

Certain foods are naturally anti-inflammatory and can help protect cells from oxidative stress, closely linked to cellular aging.

- Berries: Rich in antioxidants, berries help fight inflammation and boost immunity.

- Green Tea: Contains catechins, powerful antioxidants that reduce inflammation.

- Turmeric: The curcumin in turmeric has well-documented anti-inflammatory and antioxidant effects.

Tip: Add a handful of berries to your breakfast and a pinch of turmeric to your meals, or enjoy a cup of green tea as part of your daily routine. These small additions can significantly support your cells by reducing chronic inflammation.

3. Practice Regular Stress Management

Stress directly affects the gut, disrupting the balance of beneficial bacteria and increasing inflammation. Incorporate stress-reducing practices like meditation, deep breathing, and gentle exercise into your daily life. These habits will support gut health and reduce overall inflammation, helping your cells thrive.

Putting It All Together: A Holistic Approach to Gut and Cellular Health

Embracing gut health as the gateway to cellular vitality isn't about restrictive diets or complicated regimens. Instead, it's about nurturing your body's natural processes with sustainable, enjoyable habits. By incorporating prebiotic and probiotic foods, maintaining a high-fiber diet, reducing inflammation, and managing stress, you'll create an environment where your gut microbiome and cells can flourish.

Remember, each choice you make impacts your gut microbiome and, in turn, your cellular health. When practiced consistently, these strategies help build a strong gut barrier, support nutrient absorption, and reduce inflammation—all crucial components for longevity and a life filled with energy and well-being.

As you move forward, remember that gut health is a dynamic process. It responds to positive and harmful lifestyle choices, so minor, consistent improvements can have a lasting impact. Embracing gut health is more than just a health goal; it's a commitment to a life of vitality and resilience.

In the next chapter, we'll build upon the foundation of gut health to explore how you can protect and detoxify your cells from everyday environmental toxins. By combining these approaches, you'll be creating a powerful framework for lifelong cellular health and well-being.

CHAPTER 3: The Power of Cellular Detox – Cleansing for Optimal Function

Our modern world is filled with toxins that didn't exist even a century ago. From chemicals in household products to pollutants in the air, our cells face an uphill battle every day. These toxins can accumulate in the body, impairing cellular function and leading to fatigue, brain fog, weakened immunity, and premature aging.

Cellular detoxification, or "detox," focuses on reducing this toxic load to help our cells function at their best. In this chapter, we'll dive into practical steps to eliminate toxins from your environment, daily detox practices, and natural supplements that can support cellular health.

Identifying and Eliminating Toxins from Your Environment

Reducing toxic exposure is one of the most effective steps for cellular health. Many toxins disrupt our cells' ability to function optimally, directly affecting energy levels, mood, and even cognitive health. Let's examine some common sources of toxins and how to minimize our exposure to them.

1. Household Cleaners

Household cleaning products are often filled with chemicals that can harm our cells. Ingredients like ammonia, bleach, and synthetic fragrances release volatile organic compounds (VOCs) that can irritate the respiratory system, damage cells, and lead to inflammation.

How to Detox Your Cleaning Routine:

Switch to Natural Alternatives: Use simple, non-toxic cleaners like vinegar and baking soda. These are highly effective for most cleaning tasks and do not release harmful VOCs.

Look for Certified Products: Choose products labeled as "eco-friendly" or "certified organic." Brands like Seventh Generation and Mrs. Meyer's offer cleaner alternatives that are gentler on your home and your cells.

DIY Essential Oil Cleaner: Combine vinegar, water, and a few drops of essential oils (like tea tree oil for antibacterial properties) for a natural, effective cleaning solution.

2. Personal Care Products

Shampoos, lotions, and cosmetics often contain parabens, sulfates, and phthalates, which can disrupt cellular function by mimicking or blocking natural hormones. These toxins can accumulate, impacting cellular health and overall hormone balance.

How to Detox Your Beauty Routine:

Choose Clean Beauty Products: Look for products labeled "paraben-free," "phthalate-free," and "sulfate-free." Brands like Burt's Bees, Dr. Bronner's, and 100% Pure offer products free from these common toxins.

Read the Ingredients List: Avoid products with synthetic fragrances or colors, as these often contain harmful chemicals.

Simplify Your Routine: Sometimes, less is more. Limiting the number of products you use reduces the total toxic load on your skin and body.

3. Plastics and Food Storage

Many plastic products, especially those used for food storage, contain BPA and phthalates, which can leach into food and disrupt hormone balance. These chemicals can affect cell membranes, reducing their ability to regulate what enters and exits the cell, impacting overall cellular health.

How to Detox Your Kitchen:

- Switch to Glass or Stainless Steel Containers: Store food in glass containers to avoid exposure to plastic chemicals.

- Avoid Heating Plastics: Never microwave food in plastic containers, as heating can increase the release of harmful chemicals.

- Filter Your Water: Tap water can contain contaminants like heavy metals and chlorine. Using a high-quality water filter can reduce exposure to these toxins.

4. Indoor Air Quality

Indoor air can be surprisingly toxic, with pollutants from furniture, carpets, and air fresheners. These pollutants can impair respiratory health and cellular function, contributing to inflammation and fatigue.

How to Improve Indoor Air Quality:

- Use an Air Purifier: Invest in a high-quality air purifier, especially if you live in a city or have allergies.

- Add Indoor Plants: Plants like snake plants, spider plants, and peace lilies help naturally filter toxins from the air.

- Ventilate Regularly: Open windows whenever possible to allow fresh air to circulate and dilute indoor pollutants.

Practical Steps for Daily Detoxification

Once we've minimized exposure, the next step is actively supporting our body's detoxification systems. Our cells are equipped to handle toxins, but modern life often overwhelms these natural processes. Here are some daily practices to help your body detox more effectively.

1. Hydrate for Cellular Cleansing

Water is essential for flushing toxins out of your system. Every cell relies on adequate hydration to function correctly, and dehydration can slow down your body's natural detox processes, leading to fatigue and brain fog.

- Drink at least 8-10 Glasses a Day: Start each morning with a large glass of water to rehydrate after sleep.

- Add Lemon to Boost Detox: Lemon contains vitamin C, an antioxidant that helps neutralize toxins. Squeeze fresh lemon into your water for an added detox boost.

- Try Herbal Teas: Teas like dandelion and ginger support the liver, one of the body's primary detox organs. Drinking these in the afternoon or evening can aid in detoxification.

2. Incorporate Fiber-Rich Foods

Fiber binds to toxins and helps remove them from the body. It also supports gut health by nourishing beneficial bacteria in your microbiome, aiding digestion and immune function.

- Eat a Variety of Fiber Sources: Vegetables, fruits, legumes, and whole grains are excellent sources of fiber. Aim for at least 25-30 grams of fiber per day.

- Add Ground Flaxseed: Flaxseed is particularly effective for detoxification because it contains soluble and insoluble fiber, which supports digestion and binds toxins.

- Try Leafy Greens: Foods like kale, spinach, and arugula contain chlorophyll, which can help bind and eliminate heavy metals from the body.

3. Sweat Out Toxins

Sweating is one of the body's natural detoxification methods. Regular exercise, saunas, or hot baths can encourage sweating and promote toxin release through the skin.

- Exercise Regularly: Aim for 30 minutes of exercise that elevates your heart rate, such as brisk walking, cycling, or yoga.

- Try Infrared Saunas: Infrared saunas help detoxify at a deeper level by encouraging sweating and increasing circulation.

- Epsom Salt Baths: Epsom salts contain magnesium, which supports detoxification. A warm bath with Epsom salts can also promote relaxation and reduce stress.

4. Support Your Liver and Kidneys

The liver and kidneys are your body's primary detox organs, working tirelessly to filter out toxins. Giving them extra support can enhance your detox and overall cellular function.

- Eat Cruciferous Vegetables: Broccoli, cauliflower, and Brussels sprouts contain compounds that support liver detoxification.

- Drink Green Tea: Rich in antioxidants, green tea supports liver function and helps the body eliminate toxins.

- Limit Alcohol and Processed Foods: Alcohol and processed foods place an additional burden on the liver. Reducing these can free up your liver to focus on eliminating toxins.

Natural Supplements and Herbs to Support Cellular Detox

Certain natural supplements and herbs, in addition to lifestyle changes, can further support cellular detoxification. However, choosing supplements is essential, as some can have side effects. Always consult with a healthcare provider before adding new supplements to your routine.

1. Milk Thistle for Liver Health

Milk thistle contains silymarin, a compound that protects and supports the liver's detox functions. It can help cells regenerate after exposure to toxins and improve liver enzyme levels.

- How to Use: Look for milk thistle supplements standardized to 70-80% silymarin. Take 100-300 mg daily to support liver health.

2. Chlorella and Spirulina for Heavy Metal Detox

Chlorella and spirulina are algae that bind to heavy metals in the body, aiding in their removal. They are rich in chlorophyll and antioxidants, which can protect cells from toxin damage.

- How to Use: Start with 1-2 grams daily and gradually increase as tolerated. Choose high-quality, organic sources to avoid contamination.

3. Turmeric for Anti-Inflammatory Support

Turmeric contains curcumin, a powerful antioxidant that reduces inflammation and supports liver function. It helps the body manage oxidative stress, which often accompanies toxin exposure.

- How to Use: Take a standardized turmeric or curcumin supplement, ideally combined with black pepper to enhance absorption. 500-1000 mg daily can support detox and reduce inflammation.

4. Dandelion Root for Kidney and Liver Support

Dandelion root has been used for centuries to support liver and kidney health. It promotes bile production, which helps the liver eliminate toxins.

- How to Use: Drink dandelion tea or take a 500-1000 mg supplement daily to support detox.

Putting It All Together

Cellular detox doesn't require an expensive cleanse or a drastic lifestyle overhaul. By making small, consistent changes—like switching to non-toxic products, drinking more water, adding fiber, and incorporating supportive supplements—you can reduce your body's toxic load and give your cells the environment they need to thrive.

The power of cellular health lies in these seemingly simple actions. Each step to eliminate toxins and support your cells will bring you closer to the vibrant, energized life you envision.

As you practice these detox strategies, you're protecting your body today and investing in a healthier, more resilient future. Embrace the process and trust that these small changes, over time, will lead to profound results.

CHAPTER 4: Reclaiming Energy – From Fatigue to Vitality

Fatigue is one of the most common complaints in modern life. For many, it's an accepted part of the daily routine, whether relying on caffeine to get through the morning or feeling drained before the afternoon begins. But what if constant fatigue didn't have to be the norm?

The Power of Cellular Health aims to help you understand why you're tired and, more importantly, how to reclaim your energy. When we tackle fatigue at the cellular level, we're not just masking the symptoms—we're solving the root causes of low energy and empowering you to feel vibrant daily.

Key Causes of Low Energy and How to Address Them

Before exploring solutions, it's essential to understand the common culprits behind low energy. Many of these factors affect us daily, often without us even realizing their impact on our cellular health. Let's break down these key causes and see how they relate to cellular function.

1. Mitochondrial Dysfunction

Your cells rely on mitochondria, the tiny energy factories within each cell, to produce adenosine triphosphate (ATP)—the primary energy currency of the body. When mitochondria are working efficiently, they convert the food we eat and the oxygen we breathe into energy.

However, factors like poor diet, chronic stress, and exposure to toxins can impair mitochondrial function. When mitochondria struggle to produce energy, fatigue sets in, often leaving you feeling depleted.

Solution: Supporting mitochondrial health is crucial for sustained energy. Incorporate antioxidant-rich foods, such as berries, dark leafy greens, and nuts, to combat oxidative stress in the mitochondria.

Additionally, exercise—especially activities like brisk walking or weight training—can stimulate mitochondrial biogenesis, the process of forming new mitochondria. Regular movement helps your body create more "energy factories" to meet your daily demands.

2. Chronic Inflammation

Inflammation is a natural immune response, but when it becomes chronic, it disrupts cellular function. Chronic inflammation taxes the immune system, requiring your body to divert energy to fight off what it perceives as threats. This diversion can leave you feeling exhausted, sluggish, and foggy.

Solution: Adopt an anti-inflammatory diet to ease the burden on your immune system and support cellular energy. Foods like fatty fish, olive oil, turmeric, and ginger contain anti-inflammatory compounds that can help.

Avoid highly processed foods, sugary snacks, and refined carbohydrates, known to increase inflammation. Additionally, consider adding turmeric or ginger tea to your routine. Both spices contain natural anti-inflammatory agents that are gentle on the system.

3. Nutrient Deficiencies

Our cells require various nutrients to perform their functions. Critical nutrients like magnesium, iron, B vitamins, and CoQ10 are essential in energy production. Without enough of these nutrients, your body can't efficiently convert food into energy, leading to feelings of fatigue.

Solution: Pay attention to nutrient intake, especially if you feel tired. Include a variety of colorful vegetables, lean proteins, and whole grains in your diet. For instance, spinach, nuts, and whole grains are magnesium-rich, while lean meats and legumes provide iron.

Consult with a healthcare professional to determine if supplementation could benefit you if necessary. For example, a B-complex vitamin can support energy levels by enhancing cellular metabolism, while CoQ10 is a powerful antioxidant that directly benefits mitochondrial function.

4. Dehydration

Even mild dehydration can impair cellular function, affecting energy levels and cognitive performance. Water is essential for every biochemical reaction in the body, including those responsible for energy production. When feeling dehydrated, these processes slow down, leading to sluggishness and reduced mental clarity.

Solution:

- Make hydration a priority.

- Aim for at least 8 glasses of water daily, or more if you're active.

- Start your morning with a glass of water to rehydrate after sleep, and try adding lemon for a refreshing twist.

- Carry a water bottle with you during the day as a reminder to stay hydrated.

5. Poor Sleep Quality

Quality sleep is crucial for cellular repair and energy production. During sleep, your body undergoes various restorative processes, including cellular detoxification and the synthesis of energy-regulating hormones.

Insufficient or poor-quality sleep disrupts these processes, leaving you feeling drained the next day.

Solution:

- Practice good sleep hygiene by establishing a consistent bedtime routine.

- Avoid screen time at least an hour before bed, as blue light can interfere with melatonin production, the hormone that regulates sleep.

- Consider winding down with relaxing activities, like reading or gentle stretching, to prepare your body for rest.

- Quality sleep is one of the most effective ways to recharge your cells and support sustained energy.

Simple Lifestyle Changes to Boost Cellular Energy

Now that we've covered some fundamental causes of low energy let's explore practical lifestyle changes that support cellular energy. These changes are straightforward yet impactful, helping you create a daily routine that fosters vitality.

1. Adopt a Balanced, Energizing Diet

The food you eat is one of the most significant influences on cellular energy levels. A diet high in processed foods, sugar, and unhealthy fats burdens your cells and contributes to inflammation. In contrast, a nutrient-dense diet supports cellular health and provides a steady source of energy throughout the day.

- Prioritize Whole Foods: Opt for foods in their natural state, such as fruits, vegetables, lean proteins, and whole grains. These foods contain a wealth of vitamins, minerals, and antioxidants that support cellular health.

- Choose Low-Glycemic Carbs: High-glycemic carbohydrates, like white bread and sugary snacks, lead to energy spikes followed by crashes. Low-glycemic options like quinoa, sweet potatoes, and legumes provide a slower, more sustained release of energy.

- Include Healthy Fats: Fats are essential for energy, especially long-term energy stores. Incorporate sources like avocados, olive oil, nuts, and seeds to nourish your cells and stabilize energy levels.

2. Incorporate Regular Movement

Exercise isn't just good for physical fitness; it's a powerful tool for cellular health. Physical activity encourages mitochondria to produce energy more efficiently and stimulates the production of new mitochondria, enhancing your cells' ability to meet your energy needs.

- Engage in Aerobic Exercise: Walking, cycling, and swimming are excellent for cardiovascular health and cellular energy. Aerobic exercise increases the cell oxygen supply, which is essential for ATP production.

- Try Strength Training: Strength training, such as weight lifting, also benefits mitochondrial function and promotes muscle health, which is crucial for sustained energy. Aim for two or three weekly sessions, focusing on major muscle groups.

- Incorporate Stretching or Yoga: These practices support flexibility, reduce stress, and improve circulation—all of which benefit cellular health. Even a 10-minute stretching routine in the morning or evening can boost your energy levels.

3. Practice Mindful Breathing

Oxygen is a critical component in the production of cellular energy. Many of us breathe shallowly, especially during times of stress, limiting our oxygen intake. Mindful breathing can increase oxygen flow to the cells, enhancing cellular energy.

- Try Deep Breathing Exercises: Set aside a few minutes daily to focus on deep, slow breathing. Inhale through your nose, allowing your abdomen to rise, then exhale slowly through your mouth. This practice not only improves oxygen intake but also calms the nervous system.

- Incorporate Breathing Breaks: Throughout your day, take short breaks to focus on your breath. Even a few deep breaths can increase oxygen flow to your cells, reducing stress and boosting energy.

4. Limit Caffeine and Sugar Dependence

While caffeine and sugar offer quick energy boosts, they often lead to crashes that leave you feeling more drained than before. Over-reliance on these substances can also disrupt cellular function, as they stress the adrenal system and lead to blood sugar fluctuations.

- Gradually Reduce Intake: Instead of abruptly eliminating caffeine or sugar, gradually reduce your intake. For example, switch from sugary sodas to flavored water or herbal tea.

- Opt for Natural Energy Boosters: Try green tea, which contains moderate caffeine and provides antioxidants that support cellular health. Herbal teas like peppermint and ginger can also offer gentle energy boosts without the crash.

Nourishing Your Cells for Sustainable Energy All Day

Sustained energy requires a steady supply of nutrients that support cellular health. Let's explore some of the most potent cellular-nourishing foods and supplements that can help keep your energy levels stable and vibrant.

1. Focus on Protein for Cellular Repair and Energy

Protein is essential for cellular repair, growth, and energy production. It provides the amino acids necessary for muscle health, immune function, and cell regeneration.

- **Add Lean Proteins:** Foods like chicken, turkey, fish, tofu, and legumes provide high-quality protein. Try to include a protein source in each meal to support steady energy.

- **Consider Protein Smoothies:** If you're short on time, protein smoothies made with plant-based or whey protein powder mixed with greens and berries can offer a quick energy boost.

2. Incorporate Iron-Rich Foods for Oxygen Delivery

Iron plays a crucial role in transporting oxygen to cells. Without adequate iron, your cells can't produce energy efficiently, leading to fatigue.

- Eat Iron-Rich Foods: Include iron-rich options like lean meats, lentils, spinach, and pumpkin seeds. Pair iron sources with vitamin C (like bell peppers or oranges) to enhance absorption.

- Check Iron Levels if Necessary: If you're experiencing persistent fatigue, consider having your iron levels checked by a healthcare provider, as low iron can contribute.

3. Use Adaptogens to Support Stress Management

Adaptogens are herbs that help the body manage stress, which can indirectly benefit cellular energy. By supporting the adrenal system, adaptogens like ashwagandha, Rhodiola, and holy basil can help stabilize energy levels.

- Adaptogens to Your Routine: Add adaptogens like ashwagandha to smoothies or take them as supplements. These herbs can support resilience and sustained energy, especially during times of stress.

- Use Mindfully: Adaptogens work best when incorporated consistently but moderately. Always start with a small dose to see how your body responds.

You can transform fatigue into vitality by understanding the root causes of low energy, making small but impactful lifestyle changes, and nourishing your cells with the proper nutrients.

Cellular energy isn't just about feeling better today—it's about setting yourself up for sustained energy and well-being in the years to come. Each step you take to support your cells brings you closer to a life where you're not merely getting by, but truly thriving.

CHAPTER 5: The Essential Role of Sunlight in Cellular Health

Sunlight has been a natural source of energy, warmth, and life on Earth for centuries. But sunlight is essential to our cellular health beyond its immediate benefits.

In recent years, scientific research has revealed how sunlight impacts our cells, influencing everything from energy production in our mitochondria to hormone regulation and even our mental well-being.

Yet, in today's world, where we spend most of our time indoors, we often miss out on these benefits, depriving our cells of a critical element for optimal function.

In this chapter, we'll explore how sunlight impacts cellular and mitochondrial health, how to naturally optimize vitamin D levels and circadian rhythms, and practical strategies for safely incorporating sunlight into daily life.

How Sunlight Impacts Your Cellular and Mitochondrial Health

Sunlight is more than just a source of warmth; it provides energy and information that our cells need to function optimally. At the cellular level, sunlight directly impacts the mitochondria, the powerhouses of our cells that produce ATP (adenosine triphosphate), the body's primary energy currency. ATP is crucial for every function in the body, from muscle contraction to brain function and immune response.

1. Sunlight and Mitochondrial Efficiency

When our skin is exposed to sunlight, specifically red and near-infrared wavelengths, it stimulates mitochondrial function. This process enhances our cells' efficiency in producing ATP, giving us more energy and vitality.

Studies have shown that exposure to these wavelengths can improve mitochondrial performance, reduce oxidative stress, and support cellular repair.

For example, people who experience chronic fatigue or low energy often have compromised mitochondrial function. By incorporating regular, safe sunlight exposure, they can see improvements in energy levels because their cells produce ATP more efficiently.

This is especially beneficial for those who feel sluggish and depleted after spending long hours indoors under artificial lighting, which lacks the red and near-infrared wavelengths that natural sunlight provides.

2. Sunlight's Role in Regulating Hormones

Sunlight is also critical in regulating hormones that influence mood, sleep, and immune function. Exposure to natural light helps to stimulate the production of serotonin, a neurotransmitter associated with mood regulation.

Low levels of serotonin are linked to feelings of depression and fatigue, especially during the winter months when sunlight is scarce. Regular sunlight exposure can help elevate serotonin levels, contributing to a more positive mood and mental clarity.

Additionally, sunlight exposure in the morning triggers a rise in cortisol levels, which supports wakefulness and energy throughout the day. Conversely, exposure to blue light in the evening disrupts melatonin production, a hormone crucial for restful sleep. Understanding these natural hormonal rhythms allows us to align our habits to optimize our mood, sleep, and overall well-being.

3. Sunlight's Impact on Immune Health

Vitamin D, often called the "sunshine vitamin," is produced when the skin is exposed to UVB rays from the sun. Vitamin D plays a vital role in immune function, supporting the body's ability to fend off infections and inflammation. Low vitamin D levels are associated with a higher risk of chronic illnesses, including autoimmune diseases, cardiovascular issues, and certain cancers.

Maintaining adequate vitamin D levels can be challenging for those who frequently live indoors or in areas with limited sunlight, which may impact their immune health.

While vitamin D supplements can help, sunlight remains the most effective and natural way to boost vitamin D production, supporting overall cellular and immune health.

Optimizing Vitamin D and Circadian Rhythms Naturally

To fully harness the health benefits of sunlight, it's essential to understand how to optimize vitamin D levels and support circadian rhythms, our body's internal clock that regulates sleep, energy, and many other functions.

1. The Importance of Vitamin D for Cellular Health

Vitamin D plays an essential role in maintaining the health of your cells. Not only does it support immune function, but it also helps regulate calcium levels, which are vital for cell signaling and communication. Vitamin D receptors are found in nearly every cell in the body, meaning that adequate levels of this vitamin influence a wide range of cellular functions.

For example, studies show that people with higher vitamin D levels have better muscle function, cognitive health, and bone density.

Those with deficiencies, on the other hand, often experience fatigue, bone pain, and even weakened immunity. Vitamin D's impact on immune cells, such as T cells and macrophages, enables these cells to function effectively, protecting the body against pathogens.

How to Optimize Vitamin D Levels:

- Get Sunlight Exposure: Aim for 10-30 minutes of sunlight exposure daily, depending on your skin tone and sensitivity to sunlight. The midday sun is often the best time for vitamin D synthesis since UVB rays are strongest.

- Balance with Supplementation: If you live in a region with limited sunlight, especially during winter, consider supplementing with vitamin D3. Consult your healthcare provider to determine the right dosage based on your blood levels.

- Include Vitamin D-Rich Foods: Foods like fatty fish (salmon, mackerel), egg yolks, and fortified dairy products can also help boost vitamin D levels, although sunlight remains the most effective source.

2. Aligning with Your Circadian Rhythm

Our bodies are designed to follow natural cycles of light and dark. Disruptions to this rhythm, such as late-night screen time or irregular sleep patterns, can negatively impact cellular health, as our cells rely on these cues to regulate energy production, hormone levels, and immune function. Aligning our activities with our circadian rhythm supports cellular repair, reduces inflammation, and enhances mental clarity.

Steps to Support Your Circadian Rhythm:

- Morning Sunlight: Start your day with exposure to natural light, ideally within the first hour of waking. Morning sunlight contains more blue light, which signals your body to reduce melatonin production and increase cortisol, supporting alertness and focus.

- Avoid Artificial Light at Night: Limit exposure to blue light from screens in the evening. If this isn't possible, consider using blue-light-blocking glasses or enabling night mode on your devices.

- Establish a Consistent Sleep Schedule: Try to go to bed and wake up at the same time each day, even on weekends. This consistency reinforces your body's natural rhythm, making it easier to fall asleep and wake up feeling refreshed.

Strategies to Safely Incorporate Sun Exposure in Daily Life

While sunlight offers numerous health benefits, practicing safe sun exposure is essential to avoid the risks associated with excessive UV exposure, such as sunburn and skin damage. Here are practical ways to integrate sunlight into your routine while protecting your skin.

1. Gradual Exposure

If you're not used to spending time in the sun, start with short intervals of sun exposure and gradually increase the time as your skin adapts. This approach helps prevent sunburn and allows your body to acclimate.

For example, start with 10-15 minutes of sun exposure on your arms and legs daily, increasing the duration by a few minutes each week. If you have fair skin, stick to shorter intervals to avoid burning, while those with darker skin may need more prolonged exposure to achieve the same benefits.

2. Mindful Sun Exposure Timing

Timing is crucial when it comes to safe sun exposure. Aim for early morning or late afternoon sun, as the UV index is lower during these times, reducing the risk of sunburn. Midday sun exposure, while beneficial for vitamin D synthesis, requires extra caution due to higher UV levels.

How to Optimize Timing:

- For Vitamin D: Late morning or midday sun exposure is best, as UVB rays are more robust and effective for vitamin D production.

- For General Health: Aim for early morning sunlight exposure, lower in UVB but rich in the blue light spectrum, supporting circadian rhythm and energy.

3. Protective Measures Without Blocking Benefits

Sunscreen prevents sun damage, but excessive use can hinder vitamin D production. To balance safety and health benefits, consider using sunscreen on high-risk areas like your face and shoulders while allowing other parts of your body to be exposed for brief periods.

Tips for Sun Protection:

- Choose Broad-Spectrum Sunscreen: Look for sunscreens labeled "broad-spectrum" to protect against UVA and UVB rays, and apply as directed when exposed for extended periods.

- Wear Protective Clothing: Lightweight, long-sleeved clothing can protect your skin without blocking airflow. Hats and sunglasses also shield sensitive areas like your face and eyes.

- Use Shade Wisely: Take breaks in the shade to avoid prolonged exposure, especially during peak hours when UV radiation is most vital.

Embracing the Healing Power of Sunlight

Sunlight is one of nature's most accessible and powerful tools for supporting cellular health. From enhancing mitochondrial efficiency and regulating hormones to boosting vitamin D and aligning circadian rhythms, sunlight influences countless processes that impact how we feel, think, and function.

By approaching sun exposure mindfully, we can harness these benefits while minimizing risks, supporting a life of vitality and resilience.

With the strategies outlined in this chapter, you now have a roadmap to incorporate sunlight into your life to support and strengthen your cells. Start small, adjust as you go, and notice the changes you feel. A few minutes each day can set the foundation for healthier cells, better mood, improved immunity, and more restful sleep.

Remember, our bodies are designed to thrive harmoniously with nature's rhythms. Sunlight is a powerful ally in your journey toward cellular health—embrace it with gratitude and enjoy the transformation it brings.

CHAPTER 6: Movement and Exercise for Cell Renewal and Longevity

Physical movement is often associated with fitness goals, but its impact goes deeper than muscle tone or weight control. Regular movement and exercise are powerful tools for cellular health, directly influencing how our cells function, repair, and renew. Research continues to reveal that physical activity strengthens the body and profoundly affects cellular rejuvenation and longevity.

This chapter will explore how movement impacts your cells, rejuvenating them and providing a solid foundation for long-term health. We'll also address the challenges of fitting exercise into a busy schedule and provide tailored exercise plans to accommodate different fitness levels.

By the end, you'll have a clear path to incorporating meaningful movement into your daily routine, ensuring you can reap exercise's benefits at every stage of life.

The Science Behind Exercise and Cellular Rejuvenation

Let's start with cellular function and renewal basics to understand how movement supports cellular health. Each cell in your body is like a tiny engine that requires fuel, maintenance, and rest. Cells rely on a process called mitochondrial function to produce energy.

Mitochondria, often called the "powerhouses" of cells, convert nutrients and oxygen into ATP (adenosine triphosphate), the energy currency for your cells. As we age, mitochondrial function tends to decline, leading to reduced energy, cognitive slowdown, and other signs of aging.

How Exercise Benefits Mitochondria:

Exercise has been shown to stimulate mitochondrial biogenesis, which is how cells create new mitochondria. The more mitochondria you have, the greater your cells' energy production capabilities. A well-functioning mitochondria system means more energy at the cellular level, which translates to increased stamina, mental clarity, and overall vitality. Think of exercise as a way to "charge up" your cells and keep them functioning at their best.

Exercise and Autophagy:

Autophagy is the body's natural process of cleaning out damaged cells and regenerating new ones. This process is critical for cellular health, as it helps remove cellular debris and promotes renewal.

Exercise, particularly high-intensity and endurance training, has been shown to stimulate autophagy, kick-starting your cells' cleanup and repair processes. Regular movement ensures that cells maintain their efficiency and longevity, which plays a significant role in how we age.

Impact on Telomeres:

Telomeres are protective caps at the end of DNA strands that prevent our chromosomes from deteriorating. As we age, telomeres shorten, leading to cellular aging and reduced health.

Studies show that consistent physical activity helps maintain telomere length, effectively slowing down the aging process at the cellular level. In other words, exercise doesn't just make you feel younger; it keeps your cells younger too.

Tailored Exercise Plans for All Fitness Levels

A common pain point for many people is feeling overwhelmed by complicated fitness routines or the idea that only intense workouts yield results. However, the benefits of movement can be experienced at any fitness level, and even small amounts of activity can significantly impact cellular health.

Here, we'll break down exercise plans accessible to beginners, intermediate exercisers, and advanced athletes. No matter where you're starting from, you'll find an approach that works for you.

1. Beginner Level: Gentle Movement for Foundational Health

If you're new to exercise or have been inactive for a while, starting small is essential to building a sustainable habit. Gentle movement is just as decisive for cellular health, especially if done consistently.

- Walking: Walking is one of the simplest forms of exercise, but it has profound benefits. Aim for 20–30 minutes of brisk walking daily. Walking not only enhances mitochondrial health but also supports cardiovascular function and reduces stress. Consider breaking it up into smaller chunks if you're short on time—a few 10-minute walks throughout the day can be just as effective.

- Stretching and Flexibility Exercises: Simple stretches improve circulation and flexibility, which help nourish cells with oxygen and nutrients. Try incorporating a 10-minute stretching routine every morning or evening to help with cellular repair and rejuvenation.

- Gentle Yoga: Yoga focuses on breathing, flexibility, and low-impact movement. Poses like child's pose, downward-facing dog, and gentle twists help stimulate circulation, support lymphatic drainage, and encourage cellular detoxification.

2. Intermediate Level: Building Cellular Strength and Resilience

For those with some experience in physical activity, a moderate-intensity routine can further amplify cellular benefits. Exercises incorporating strength and endurance are particularly valuable for mitochondrial health at this level.

- Strength Training: Aim to incorporate strength training exercises twice a week. Resistance bands, body-weight exercises like squats and lunges, or light weights are excellent for beginners. Strength training stimulates muscle growth and increases mitochondrial density, supporting energy production.

- Interval Training: High-intensity interval training (HIIT) involves alternating short bursts of intense exercise with rest periods. For example, 30 seconds of fast-paced jogging or jumping jacks followed by 30 seconds of rest, repeated for 10 minutes. HIIT is particularly effective in stimulating mitochondrial biogenesis and autophagy, which supports cellular repair.

- Swimming or Cycling: Low-impact aerobic activities like swimming and cycling are easy on the joints and provide excellent cardiovascular and mitochondrial benefits. Aim for 20–30 minutes of these activities 2–3 times weekly to support cellular health and improve endurance.

3. Advanced Level: Optimizing Cellular Performance

For those who are more experienced, a higher-intensity routine can push cellular health to peak levels. Advanced exercisers can benefit from incorporating aerobic, anaerobic, and recovery-focused exercises.

- Heavy Strength Training: For those comfortable with weight lifting, heavier resistance can stimulate muscle fibers and mitochondrial activity, supporting both strength and endurance at the cellular level. Focus on compound movements like deadlifts, bench presses, and squats.

- High-Intensity Interval Training (HIIT): Advanced HIIT routines—such as Tabata (20 seconds of high-intensity exercise followed by 10 seconds of rest for 4 minutes)—can effectively promote autophagy and mitochondrial health. Perform this 2–3 times per week to maximize cellular regeneration.

- Mindful Recovery: Advanced exercisers benefit greatly from recovery practices. Stretching, foam rolling, and breathwork help reduce inflammation and support the body's cellular repair processes. These activities ensure that cells are restored and ready for the next challenge.

How to Incorporate Movement into a Busy Lifestyle

One of the most common challenges people face is finding the time to exercise. Busy lifestyles, long work hours, and family responsibilities can make regular exercise seem unattainable.

However, you don't need to carve out hours each day to experience the benefits of movement. Here are practical ways to incorporate exercise into your daily routine without disrupting your schedule.

1. Start Small and Build Consistency

Rather than aiming for long sessions, focus on short bursts of activity throughout the day. Studies show that even 10–15 minutes of exercise can positively impact mitochondrial health and energy levels. Try doing short sessions multiple times daily—such as a 10-minute walk after lunch and another in the evening.

- Example: Set a timer to stand up and move every hour. Walk around your office, do a few stretches, or practice deep breathing. These short breaks can increase blood flow, boost energy, and help keep your cells functioning optimally.

2. Incorporate Movement into Daily Tasks

Adding movement to everyday tasks is a simple yet effective way to stay active. Look for opportunities to move as part of your routine, turning daily activities into exercise without needing a designated workout time.

- Take the Stairs: Whenever possible, choose stairs over elevators. This quick burst of movement can increase your heart rate and support mitochondrial function.

- Stand While Working: If your job involves extended periods of sitting, consider a standing desk. Standing engages more muscles than sitting and improves circulation, which benefits cellular health.

- Active Commuting: If possible, walk or bike to work instead of driving. If that's not an option, try parking further away from your destination or getting off public transport a stop early to add a few extra minutes of walking.

3. Make It a Family Affair

Incorporating exercise as a family activity makes it easier to stay consistent and encourages a healthy lifestyle for everyone. Outdoor activities like hiking, biking, or playing sports together provide meaningful exercise while creating quality time.

- Example: Plan weekend hikes or bike rides with family or friends. These activities are enjoyable and boost cardiovascular health, improve mitochondrial function, and provide fresh air, which is essential for cellular respiration.

4. Use Technology to Stay Accountable

Wearable fitness trackers and mobile apps can help you track movement, set goals, and even receive reminders to stay active throughout the day. Many apps allow you to log different types of activity, track your progress, and celebrate milestones, which can be motivating.

- Example: Set a daily step goal with a fitness tracker and aim to reach it by the end of the day. Even small goals, like reaching 5,000 or 10,000 steps, encourage consistent movement, which benefits cellular health.

5. Find Activities You Enjoy

The best exercise is the one you look forward to doing. Experiment with different types of movement until you find what feels suitable for you, whether it's dancing, swimming, yoga, or something else. Enjoyable activities are more accessible to stick with, ensuring that exercise becomes a sustainable habit.

Embrace Movement as Part of Your Cellular Health Journey

Exercise doesn't have to be complicated or time-consuming to be effective. Consistent, enjoyable movement at any fitness level can profoundly affect your cellular health.

By understanding the science behind how exercise impacts your cells, tailoring a plan to your needs, and finding ways to incorporate movement into a busy lifestyle, you're setting yourself up for a life of vitality and resilience.

The path to longevity and cellular health is as much about building habits as it is about understanding science. Each step, each stretch, and each lift contributes to a healthier cellular environment that supports your energy, mental clarity, and overall well-being. Embrace movement as a vital part of your journey, and trust that these small actions will create lasting benefits that you'll carry with you at every age.

CHAPTER 7: Cellular Nutrition – Eating to Fuel Longevity

The food we eat is more than just fuel—it's information that shapes our health at the cellular level. Every bite we take influences how our cells function, repair, and respond to aging. Our diets are pivotal in our vitality, resilience, and longevity.

In this chapter, we'll explore how to embrace balanced nutrition to support cellular health, focusing on healthy fats, carbohydrates, and proteins while avoiding inflammatory foods. We'll also look at how to create easy, nourishing meal plans that can help you unlock the potential of your cells.

Embracing Healthy Fats, Carbs, and Proteins for Cellular Health

Each macronutrient—fats, carbohydrates, and proteins—has a distinct role in cellular health. Understanding how to balance these in your diet is key to giving your cells the fuel they need to thrive.

1. Healthy Fats: Essential for Cell Membrane Integrity and Energy

Fats are crucial for cellular health. They form the structure of every cell membrane, allowing cells to maintain their integrity and communicate effectively. The right kinds of fats can help protect cells, while the wrong ones can create inflammation and damage cellular function.

Examples of Healthy Fats:

Omega-3 Fatty Acids: In fatty fish (like salmon, sardines, and mackerel), chia seeds, and flaxseeds, omega-3s help reduce inflammation at the cellular level. They're also known to improve cell membrane flexibility, which allows cells to absorb nutrients and expel waste more efficiently.

- Monounsaturated Fats: These fats, found in foods like olive oil, avocados, and nuts, support cardiovascular health and provide steady energy to cells.

- Saturated Fats from Clean Sources: Contrary to some dietary myths, saturated fats from quality sources like coconut oil and grass-fed meats can support hormone production and cellular energy when consumed in moderation.

- Incorporating Healthy Fats: If you're new to incorporating these fats, use extra virgin olive oil as a salad dressing or cook with avocado oil. Add chia seeds to smoothies or yogurt, and include a serving of fatty fish in your diet twice a week. These small steps will help ensure your cells are supported with high-quality fats.

- Avoiding Unhealthy Fats: Processed oils such as soybean, canola, and sunflower oils are high in omega-6 fatty acids, which can promote inflammation when consumed excessively. These oils are often found in processed foods and should be avoided or minimized as much as possible to protect cellular health.

2. Carbohydrates: Fueling Cells While Avoiding Spikes

Carbohydrates provide energy to cells, but not all carbs are created equal. Simple carbohydrates, like refined sugars and white flour, can cause spikes in blood sugar and insulin, leading to cellular stress and inflammation. In contrast, complex carbohydrates provide steady energy without overwhelming the body's systems.

Examples of Beneficial Carbohydrates:

Whole Grains: Quinoa, farro, and brown rice are rich in fiber, vitamins, and minerals. They break down slowly, providing a steady release of glucose for cells to use as fuel.

- Vegetables and Fruits: Leafy greens, cruciferous vegetables, and berries are high in antioxidants, which protect cells from oxidative stress. These foods also contain fiber, which helps stabilize blood sugar levels.

- Legumes: Beans, lentils, and chickpeas are nutrient-dense and provide protein and fiber, making them excellent for cellular energy.

- Incorporating Healthy Carbs: Start by swapping out refined grains for whole grains. For example, replace white rice with quinoa or brown rice. Use sweet potatoes instead of bread for breakfast or a snack. These nutrient-dense carbs provide fiber and micronutrients that support cellular health.

- Avoiding Simple Carbs: Foods with high sugar content, like pastries, sugary cereals, and sodas, can spike blood sugar and insulin levels. Over time, these fluctuations increase the risk of inflammation and oxidative stress, impairing cellular function.

3. Proteins: Building Blocks for Cellular Repair and Maintenance

Protein is essential for building, repairing, and maintaining cellular structures. Every cell in your body needs amino acids from protein to support its functions, especially in tissues that require frequent renewal, like muscles, skin, and organs.

Examples of High-Quality Protein Sources:

- Lean Meats and Fish: Grass-fed beef, chicken, and wild-caught fish provide high-quality protein without added hormones or antibiotics. Fish is also a great source of omega-3s, making it doubly beneficial.

- Plant-Based Proteins: For those looking to reduce animal protein intake, options like lentils, chickpeas, and tofu provide essential amino acids.

- Eggs and Dairy: Eggs are an excellent source of protein and choline, which supports brain health. Look for pasture-raised eggs and dairy for higher nutrient quality.

- Incorporating Protein: Aim to include a source of protein with every meal. This doesn't have to be complicated—a handful of nuts with breakfast grilled chicken or tofu with lunch, and a piece of salmon for dinner. Protein also helps stabilize blood sugar levels, which protects cellular function.

- Avoiding Processed Proteins: Processed meats like bacon, sausages, and deli meats contain preservatives and additives that can increase oxidative stress. Limit these foods to avoid exposing your cells to unnecessary toxins.

The Impact of Sugar, Processed Foods, and Inflammation on Cells

To achieve optimal cellular health, it's essential to understand the impact of sugar, processed foods, and inflammation on your body. These elements can particularly damage cells, accelerate aging, and lead to chronic conditions.

1. Sugar and Glycation

Consuming sugar can bind to proteins and fats in your body in a process known as glycation. Glycation produces harmful compounds called advanced glycation end-products (AGEs), which can damage cellular structures and contribute to aging, inflammation, and chronic diseases.

- Example: A study showed that individuals with diets high in added sugars had higher levels of AGEs, which can damage collagen and contribute to wrinkles and joint stiffness. Reducing added sugar intake can protect cellular structures and potentially slow down visible signs of aging.

- Reducing Sugar: Start by eliminating sugary drinks and limiting desserts. Opt for natural sweeteners like stevia or enjoy fruits like berries, which provide sweetness and antioxidants that protect cells.

2. Processed Foods and Inflammatory Ingredients

Processed foods often contain artificial additives, preservatives, and trans fats, which contribute to inflammation. Chronic inflammation is detrimental to cells, as it keeps the immune system in a heightened state, which can lead to cellular damage over time.

- Example: Many fast foods contain trans fats, which increase inflammatory markers in the body. Studies have shown that regular consumption of trans fats can lead to increased oxidative stress and cellular damage, especially in blood vessels.

- Reducing Processed Foods: Limit your intake of packaged snacks, fast foods, and frozen meals. Preparing meals at home gives you control over the ingredients, allowing you to choose foods that support, rather than harm, your cellular health.

3. Oxidative Stress and Inflammation

Oxidative stress occurs when the body's free radicals and antioxidants are imbalanced. Free radicals can damage cells, leading to aging and disease. Antioxidants help neutralize these free radicals, reducing cellular stress and inflammation.

Example: Foods high in antioxidants, like blueberries, spinach, and green tea, provide a natural defense against oxidative stress. Incorporating these foods into your diet regularly can help protect cells from damage.

Easy-to-Follow Meal Plans for Optimal Cell Function

A meal plan doesn't need to be restrictive or overly complicated to support cellular health. Here are some examples of balanced meals that incorporate healthy fats, proteins, and complex carbs to nourish your cells and sustain energy throughout the day.

Sample Meal Plan for Cellular Health

Breakfast:

- Avocado Toast on Whole-Grain Bread with a Poached Egg

Provides a balance of healthy fats from avocado, protein from the egg, and fiber from whole-grain bread. This combination stabilizes blood sugar and fuels cells for the morning.

- Green Smoothie with Spinach, Chia Seeds, Blueberries, and Unsweetened Almond Milk

Packed with antioxidants and fiber, this smoothie helps combat oxidative stress and provides long-lasting energy.

Lunch:

- Quinoa Salad with Grilled Salmon, Mixed Greens, and Olive Oil Dressing

Quinoa offers complex carbs and protein, while salmon provides omega-3 fatty acids. Olive oil adds healthy monounsaturated fats that support cell membrane health.

- Side of Steamed Broccoli and Carrots

These veggies provide fiber and antioxidants that aid in cellular repair and detoxification.

Snack:

- Handful of Almonds and Fresh Berries

Almonds offer monounsaturated fats and protein, while berries provide a low-sugar source of antioxidants.

Dinner:

- Grilled Chicken Breast with Sweet Potatoes and Roasted Brussels Sprouts

Chicken provides lean protein, while sweet potatoes offer fiber and complex carbs. Brussels sprouts are rich in sulfur compounds that support detoxification.

- Herbal Tea (like Chamomile or Ginger)

Helps with digestion and reduces inflammation, supporting the cells' nighttime recovery.

Tips for Making the Meal Plan Work for You

- Prepare in Batches: At the beginning of the week, prepare grains, proteins, and vegetables in batches. This makes it easy to assemble balanced meals without much hassle.

- Experiment with Spices: Use spices like turmeric, ginger, and garlic, which have anti-inflammatory properties and can add flavor to meals without relying on processed sauces.

- Focus on Whole Foods: As a general rule, the fewer ingredients a food has, the better it is for your cells. Choose whole, unprocessed foods whenever possible.

Embracing Cellular Nutrition for Long-Term Health

By embracing a diet rich in healthy fats, proteins, and carbohydrates and reducing sugar and processed foods, you're giving your cells the nourishment they need to function at their best. Cellular nutrition isn't about perfection—it's about making conscious choices that support your body's natural processes.

Over time, these choices add up, enhancing energy, slowing aging, and supporting long-term health. By following the guidance in this chapter, you're on the path to a healthier, more resilient life powered by the foundational strength of your cells.

CHAPTER 8: Healthy Fats and Oils – Rejuvenating Your Cells

The types of fats we consume play a crucial role in our journey to support cellular health and longevity. For decades, fats have been demonized as the culprits behind weight gain and heart disease. However, emerging research reveals that not all fats are created equal.

In fact, certain fats are essential for optimal health and, when chosen wisely, can support cellular function, boost energy levels, and improve mental clarity. This chapter will explore why healthy fats are vital to cellular health, identify the oils to avoid, and guide you in choosing the best fats to rejuvenate your body from the inside out.

Understanding the Importance of Healthy Fats

Healthy fats are indispensable to our cells' structure and function. Every cell in our body is enclosed by a lipid (fat) bilayer, a membrane that protects the cell while allowing it to communicate with its surroundings. This membrane, made up primarily of fats, plays a crucial role in nutrient absorption, waste elimination, and maintaining fluid balance within the cell. The quality of the fats we consume directly influences the integrity and function of this cellular membrane.

Healthy fats support various aspects of well-being, including:

- Mental Clarity and Cognitive Function: Our brains are nearly 60% fat, and essential fatty acids—particularly omega-3s—are necessary for memory, focus, and overall cognitive health.

- Hormone Production: Fats are critical in producing hormones that regulate mood and metabolism.

- Energy Levels: Fats provide a long-lasting source of energy, as they metabolize more slowly than carbohydrates. This results in sustained energy without blood sugar spikes and crashes.

- Anti-Inflammatory Effects: Certain healthy fats, such as those rich in omega-3 fatty acids, have potent anti-inflammatory effects, essential for reducing cellular inflammation and maintaining cellular health over time.

Why Fat Quality Matters

Healthy fats can support the body's anti-inflammatory processes, reduce oxidative stress, and enhance cellular resilience. Conversely, consuming low-quality or damaged fats can contribute to inflammation, oxidative stress, and cellular dysfunction. This distinction is especially relevant in our current food environment, where processed and artificial fats are pervasive.

For example, many processed foods contain chemically altered trans fats to increase shelf life.

However, trans fats have been shown to increase the risk of heart disease, impair cellular communication, and contribute to systemic inflammation. Understanding and choosing the right fats can nourish our cells and protect our health from the inside out.

Common Cooking Oils to Avoid and What to Use Instead

The oils we choose in our kitchens can either support cellular health or work against it. Some oils are prone to oxidation, which occurs when they're exposed to heat and air.

This oxidation process creates free radicals—unstable molecules that can damage cellular structures, contribute to inflammation, and accelerate aging. To make the best choices for your health, it's essential to recognize which oils to avoid and which to prioritize.

Oils to Avoid

- Vegetable Oils (Soybean, Corn, and Canola Oil)

When consumed, these oils are often highly processed and refined, making them more prone to oxidation and inflammation. Vegetable oils also contain high levels of omega-6 fatty acids, which, while essential in small amounts, can promote inflammation when consumed in excess. Most Western diets already contain a high ratio of omega-

6 to omega-3, contributing to an imbalance promoting cellular inflammation.

- Why Avoid: Vegetable oils undergo extensive processing, including chemical extraction and high-heat refinement, which degrades their quality and makes them more susceptible to oxidation.

- Alternative: Replace vegetable oils with healthier options such as olive or avocado oil, which is rich in monounsaturated fats that support heart health and reduce inflammation.

Margarine and Shortening

Margarine and shortening were once popular alternatives to butter, but they're often made with hydrogenated oils, creating trans fats. Trans fats can disrupt cell membranes, interfere with normal cellular function, and increase the risk of cardiovascular disease.

- Why Avoid: Trans fats are detrimental to heart health and cellular function and have been associated with an increased risk of chronic diseases.

- Alternative: Choose grass-fed butter or ghee, which contain healthy saturated fats and are more stable at high heat.

Refined Coconut Oil

Coconut oil can be beneficial in its unrefined state, as it contains medium-chain triglycerides (MCTs) metabolized efficiently for energy. However, refined coconut oil undergoes bleaching and deodorizing, which strips it of its beneficial properties and can introduce harmful chemicals.

- Why Avoid: Refined coconut oil loses much of its nutritional value and may contain residues from processing.

- Alternative: If you prefer coconut oil, use unrefined, virgin coconut oil, as it retains its natural MCT content and is more beneficial for cellular health.

Grapeseed Oil

Although grapeseed oil is sometimes marketed as a "healthy" option, it contains high omega-6 fatty acids and is prone to oxidation. It's often extracted through chemical processes that can introduce residues and degrade the oil's quality.

- Why Avoid: High omega-6 content and susceptibility to oxidation make grapeseed oil a less-than-ideal choice.

- Alternative: Opt for oils with a better balance of omega-3 to omega-6 fats, like extra-virgin olive oil.

Oils to Embrace

- Extra-virgin olive oil (EVOO) is rich in monounsaturated fats, particularly oleic acid, which has been shown to reduce inflammation and support heart health. EVOO also contains antioxidants, like polyphenols, which protect cells from oxidative damage.

- How to Use: It is ideal for low—to medium-heat cooking and drizzling over salads, vegetables, or pasta.

- Benefits for Cellular Health: Olive oil's antioxidants protect cell membranes and reduce oxidative stress, while its healthy fats support cell structure and function.

Avocado Oil

Avocado oil is high in monounsaturated fats and has a high smoke point, making it suitable for various cooking methods. It also contains vitamin E, a powerful antioxidant that supports skin health and cellular resilience.

- How to Use: Suitable for high-heat cooking, including frying, roasting, and grilling.

- Benefits for Cellular Health: Avocado oil's stability at high temperatures makes it a safe option for cooking, while its nutrient profile supports anti-inflammatory and antioxidant activity in cells.

Flaxseed Oil

Flaxseed oil is one of the richest plant sources of omega-3 fatty acids, which are essential for brain health, reducing inflammation, and supporting cellular membranes. However, flaxseed oil is delicate and should not be heated, as it's prone to oxidation.

- How to Use: Flaxseed oil can be used as a finishing oil, adding it to smoothies, salads, or oatmeal.

- Benefits for Cellular Health: Omega-3s are vital for brain function, hormone balance, and reducing cellular inflammation.

Walnut Oil

Walnut oil contains omega-3 and omega-6 fatty acids, providing a balanced profile supporting brain and heart health. While it's not heat-stable, walnut oil is excellent for cold applications.

- How to Use: Ideal for salad dressings, drizzling over roasted vegetables, or incorporating into dips.

- Benefits for Cellular Health: The omega-3 content helps balance inflammation, while its antioxidants support cellular resilience.

How Changing Your Fats Can Boost Mental and Physical Vitality

Swapping unhealthy fats for beneficial ones can bring about noticeable changes in your energy, cognitive function, and overall well-being. Here's how these changes work on a cellular level.

1. Enhanced Brain Function

Healthy fats, particularly omega-3 fatty acids, are essential for cognitive health. DHA (docosahexaenoic acid), an omega-3 fat found in fish and algae oils, is a major component of brain tissue. Adequate DHA intake has been linked to improved memory, focus, and mood, as well as reduced risk of neurodegenerative diseases.

- Example: Adding omega-3-rich foods like flaxseed oil, walnuts, or fish can support brain function and improve symptoms of brain fog or mental fatigue.

- Practical Tip: Incorporate salmon or chia seeds into your meals several times a week to naturally increase your omega-3 intake.

2. Reduced Inflammation and Improved Cellular Resilience

Consuming anti-inflammatory fats like those in olive oil, avocado, and fatty fish can help reduce inflammation on a cellular level. Inflammation significantly contributes to cellular aging, so by reducing it, you're actively supporting your cells' longevity and function.

- Example: People who switch from a diet high in refined vegetable oils to one rich in monounsaturated fats often report reduced joint pain, improved digestion, and better energy levels.

- Practical Tip: Use avocado oil for cooking and olive oil for dressings to build anti-inflammatory, cell-supportive fats into your daily meals.

3. Long-Lasting Energy and Satiety

Healthy fats provide sustained energy without causing blood sugar spikes, making them ideal for maintaining steady energy levels throughout the day. Unlike refined carbs, fats metabolize slowly, keeping you satisfied and reducing the likelihood of mid-day energy crashes.

- Example: Starting your day with an avocado or a handful of nuts for breakfast can provide lasting energy and help you avoid cravings.

- Practical Tip: To increase your healthy fat intake in the morning, add a tablespoon of flaxseed oil to your morning smoothie or sprinkle chia seeds on your yogurt.

4. Improved Skin Health

The quality of the fats you consume can directly impact the health and appearance of your skin. Omega-3s, monounsaturated fats, and antioxidants in healthy oils keep skin hydrated, resilient, and better to protect itself from environmental damage.

- Example: People who incorporate olive oil or omega-3-rich foods into their diet often notice more hydrated, glowing skin.

- Practical Tip: Use extra-virgin olive oil in dressings and dips to give your skin a daily boost of hydration and protection.

Choosing the right fats isn't about restrictive diets or complex nutrition rules; it's about nourishing your body in a way that supports cellular health and longevity.

By replacing harmful oils with healthy, nutrient-rich fats, you're actively supporting your cells' structure, communication, and resilience. Over time, these small changes can significantly improve your mental clarity, energy, and overall sense of well-being.

Remember, the path to optimal health begins with the choices you make every day. By embracing healthy fats, you're giving your body the fuel to thrive at every level. Let these changes empower you to live a life of vitality and resilience from your cells up.

CHAPTER 9: Collagen and Protein – Building Blocks for Cellular Repair

Regarding cellular health, collagen, and protein are among the most crucial elements you can incorporate into your lifestyle. They serve as the foundational building blocks your body uses for cellular repair, regeneration, and longevity.

By understanding the role of collagen and protein in cellular health and knowing how to choose suitable sources and integrate them into your daily routine, you can enhance your vitality, protect against the visible and internal signs of aging, and support your body's natural repair processes.

In this chapter, we'll explore the importance of collagen and protein, practical ways to select suitable sources, and daily strategies to maximize their benefits for long-lasting cellular health.

The Role of Collagen in Cellular Health and Anti-Aging

What is Collagen?

Collagen is the most abundant protein in our bodies, providing structure and strength to our skin, bones, muscles, tendons, and ligaments.

As we age, however, our body's natural production of collagen declines, which can lead to wrinkles, joint pain, and a general decrease in skin elasticity and resilience. Collagen is essential for maintaining youthful skin and supporting cellular health at a deeper level, as it helps repair damaged cells and keeps tissues strong and flexible.

Collagen is often likened to a "scaffold" for our cells. It forms the matrix that holds everything together and helps maintain the integrity of our body's tissues. By replenishing collagen, we give our cells the support they need to function optimally, whether that's for keeping skin smooth or ensuring bones and joints remain resilient and robust.

How Collagen Supports Anti-Aging and Cellular Repair

Collagen contributes to cellular repair and anti-aging in several ways:

- Skin Elasticity and Hydration: Collagen is essential for maintaining skin elasticity and hydration. When collagen levels decline, skin begins to sag, wrinkle, and lose its youthful glow. By supporting collagen production, you help maintain a vibrant appearance.

- Joint Health and Mobility: Collagen provides cushioning for joints, reducing friction and helping prevent the wear and tear that can lead to arthritis or joint pain. Studies have shown that collagen supplements may help reduce joint pain and improve mobility, which is essential for aging adults who want to stay active and pain-free.

- Cellular Regeneration and Wound Healing: Collagen plays a key role in wound healing by promoting the regeneration of damaged cells.

This is why it's often recommended after surgeries or injuries to speed up recovery.

How to Incorporate Collagen into Your Diet

While the body can produce collagen independently, the process slows down as we age, so supplementing collagen can be particularly beneficial. Here are some practical ways to boost your collagen levels:

- Collagen Supplements: Collagen supplements come in various forms, such as powders, capsules, and liquids. Look for hydrolyzed collagen, which is broken down into smaller peptides that the body can more easily absorb. Start with a dose of around 10 grams daily, mixing it into your coffee, smoothie, or oatmeal.

- Bone Broth: Bone broth is a natural source of collagen, rich in amino acids like glycine and proline, which are essential for collagen synthesis. Try incorporating a cup of bone broth into your diet a few times a week, or use it as a base for soups and stews.

- Vitamin C-Rich Foods: Vitamin C is essential for collagen synthesis, as it helps link amino acids together to form collagen. Including foods rich in vitamin C, such as oranges, strawberries, and bell peppers, can boost your body's natural collagen production.

How to Choose the Right Protein Sources for Longevity

Protein is the foundation of cellular health, providing the amino acids necessary for building and repairing cells, tissues, enzymes, and hormones. Choosing high-quality protein sources is crucial to supporting cellular repair, maintaining muscle mass, and promoting longevity. However, not all proteins are created equal, and selecting the right ones can affect how your body functions and ages.

Complete vs. Incomplete Proteins

Proteins are made up of amino acids, some of which are "essential," meaning our bodies can't produce them independently and must obtain them from food. Complete proteins contain all nine essential amino acids, while incomplete proteins lack one or more. Complete proteins are ideal for cellular health, ensuring your body has the amino acids for optimal function.

- Animal-Based Complete Proteins: Sources include meat, poultry, fish, eggs, and dairy products. These proteins are generally more accessible for the body to absorb and utilize fully.

- Plant-Based Complete Proteins: Some plant sources, like quinoa, soy, and chia seeds, are complete proteins and can be great options for vegetarians or vegans.

Combining incomplete proteins can help ensure a complete amino acid profile for those following a plant-based diet. For example, pairing beans with rice or lentils with whole grains provides all essential amino acids.

Prioritizing Lean Proteins for Cellular Health

Choosing lean proteins, particularly those low in saturated fats, supports cellular health by reducing inflammation and avoiding the buildup of toxins that can come from consuming processed or fatty meats.

Here are some recommended protein sources for longevity:

- Fish: Rich in omega-3 fatty acids, fish like salmon, sardines, and mackerel provide high-quality protein and anti-inflammatory benefits, making them ideal for cellular repair.

- Poultry: Skinless chicken and turkey are excellent sources of lean protein, low in saturated fat, and easily digestible.

- Eggs: Eggs are a complete protein source and contain nutrients like choline, which supports brain health and cellular membrane integrity.

- Legumes: Beans, lentils, and peas are high in protein and fiber, making them great for digestive health and cellular detoxification.

- Nuts and Seeds: Almonds, chia seeds, and pumpkin seeds offer protein and healthy fats, which support cell membrane health.

Protein Timing and Distribution

For optimal protein synthesis and cell repair, it's not just about how much protein you consume, but also when and how you distribute it throughout the day. Research suggests that spreading protein intake evenly across meals can help maximize muscle maintenance and repair.

For example, if you aim for 60 grams of protein daily, try to have 20 grams at breakfast, 20 grams at lunch, and 20 grams at dinner. This consistent intake allows your body to utilize amino acids more effectively, which supports continuous cellular repair and growth.

Daily Strategies to Support Protein Synthesis and Cell Repair

Incorporating daily habits that support protein synthesis and cellular repair can significantly enhance your health and longevity. Here are some strategies to help you make the most of the protein and collagen in your diet:

1. Pair Protein with Physical Activity

Physical activity, especially resistance training and weight-bearing exercises, stimulates protein synthesis and helps maintain muscle mass, which is critical for aging gracefully. These exercises enhance muscle repair and cellular regeneration when paired with protein consumption.

- Examples of Resistance Exercises: Bodyweight exercises like squats, lunges, and push-ups, as well as weightlifting or resistance band workouts, are all excellent for promoting cellular health and protein synthesis.

- Post-Workout Protein: After exercise, aim to consume 20-30 grams of protein within an hour to maximize recovery and support muscle repair.

2. Prioritize Protein at Breakfast

Starting your day with protein sets the tone for sustained energy and supports muscle repair. Although breakfast is often a carb-heavy meal, adding protein can stabilize blood sugar, reduce cravings, and improve mental clarity.

- Breakfast Ideas: Try Greek yogurt with chia seeds, a smoothie with protein powder, or eggs with spinach and avocado.

3. Reduce Processed Foods

Processed foods are often high in unhealthy fats, additives, and sugars, contributing to inflammation and hindering protein synthesis. To support cellular function, stick to whole, unprocessed foods as much as possible, focusing on fresh vegetables, lean proteins, and healthy fats.

4. Stay Hydrated

Hydration is essential for protein synthesis and nutrient transport within cells. Dehydration can slow down protein metabolism, reducing the effectiveness of the protein you consume. Aim to drink at least eight glasses of water daily, adjusting based on your activity level.

5. Incorporate Key Nutrients for Protein Synthesis

Certain nutrients play a critical role in protein synthesis and cellular repair:

- Vitamin C: Important for collagen production and tissue repair. Include foods like oranges, strawberries, and bell peppers in your diet

- Magnesium: Supports muscle function and protein synthesis. Found in leafy greens, nuts, and whole grains.

- Zinc: This mineral is important for tissue repair and immune health. Foods like oysters, beef, and pumpkin seeds are rich in zinc.

Practical Tips for Lasting Results

Sticking to these habits can initially feel overwhelming, but creating a sustainable routine that fits your lifestyle is the goal. Here are a few tips for making these protein and collagen-supporting practices a seamless part of your daily life:

- Prep in Advance: Prepare protein-rich snacks and meals in advance to avoid reaching for processed foods. Boil eggs, portion out Greek yogurt, or make protein smoothies that you can grab on the go.

- Keep Supplements Handy: If you're using collagen or protein powders, keep them easily accessible, whether at home or in the office, so you can mix them into drinks or meals as needed.

- Track Your Progress: Over time, notice changes in your energy levels, skin, and joint health. Minor improvements can motivate you to stay consistent.

- Adjust as Needed: Your protein needs may change with your activity level, age, and goals. Check-in regularly to ensure you're meeting your body's requirements.

Embracing the Power of Protein and Collagen for Cellular Health

Collagen and protein aren't just about building muscle or keeping your skin smooth—they're integral to cellular health and vital in keeping you vibrant, resilient, and active throughout your life.

By prioritizing high-quality protein sources, supporting collagen production, and incorporating these daily strategies, you're investing in a foundation of health that supports your cells, organs, and body systems.

As you incorporate these practices, remember that cellular health is a journey. By taking steps to support protein synthesis and cellular repair, you're empowering your body to age gracefully, recover from stress and damage, and maintain a quality of life that allows you to truly thrive.

CHAPTER 10: Gut Repair and Immune Strengthening Through Smart Carbs

When we think of carbohydrates, they're often associated with quick energy or foods to avoid on restrictive diets. But when chosen wisely, carbs can be a powerful ally for cellular health, gut repair, and immune strength.

The right kinds of carbohydrates fuel the gut microbiome, enhance nutrient absorption, and provide a stable energy source. This chapter explores how specific carbohydrates support your cells, boost immunity, and play a crucial role in your body's healing processes.

How Carbohydrates Support Gut and Cellular Health

Carbohydrates have a significant role in cellular health and immunity. Complex carbohydrates, rich in fiber and resistant starch, act as prebiotics, feeding the beneficial bacteria in our gut. These friendly microbes are vital for breaking down food, producing essential nutrients, and regulating immune function. They also contribute to the health of our gut lining, which acts as a barrier to pathogens and toxins.

The link between gut health and immunity is well-established. Approximately 70% of our immune system resides in the gut, meaning that supporting the gut microbiome is one of the most effective ways to boost immune strength.

When beneficial bacteria thrive, they help outcompete harmful microbes and prevent inflammation that can weaken immunity.

Additionally, a diverse and well-nourished microbiome contributes to the integrity of the gut lining, which stops toxins from entering the bloodstream—a process known as "leaky gut" when it fails.

Here's how the right carbohydrates contribute to this process:

- Feed Beneficial Bacteria: Complex carbs found in vegetables, whole grains, and legumes are broken down slowly and serve as food for beneficial bacteria in the gut. As bacteria ferment these fibers, they produce short-chain fatty acids (SCFAs) like butyrate, which reduce inflammation, protect the gut lining, and enhance immune function.

- Stabilize Blood Sugar: Unlike simple sugars, which cause blood sugar spikes and crashes, complex carbs provide a steady energy source that supports the cells' metabolic processes. When blood sugar is stable, cells can focus on repair and regeneration rather than managing the effects of fluctuating glucose levels.

- Reduce Inflammation: Chronic inflammation is linked to a weakened immune system and cellular aging. Complex carbs, rich in antioxidants and phytonutrients, help reduce inflammation by neutralizing free radicals and supporting detoxification pathways.

- Aid in Nutrient Absorption: The fermentation process in the gut, fueled by complex carbs, aids in the absorption of nutrients that are essential for cellular function, including vitamins, minerals, and amino acids.

Choosing the Right Carbs for Optimal Immune Support

Not all carbs are created equal. Focusing on fiber-rich, low-glycemic carbohydrates is key when supporting gut health and immunity. Here's a guide to selecting carbs that benefit your cells and immune system:

1. Vegetables Rich in Fiber and Antioxidants

Vegetables are among the best sources of complex carbohydrates. They contain fiber, vitamins, and antioxidants, supporting cellular health, immune function, and detoxification.

- Examples: Sweet potatoes, carrots, broccoli, cauliflower, and spinach.

- Benefits: These vegetables are high in fiber, feed beneficial bacteria, and provide many phytonutrients that combat inflammation and oxidative stress.

2. Whole Grains for Steady Energy

Whole grains such as quinoa, brown rice, and oats are nutrient-dense and contain a mix of soluble and insoluble fiber, which helps maintain gut health.

- Examples: Quinoa, brown rice, oats, barley.

- Benefits: Whole grains support balanced blood sugar levels for cellular repair and immune resilience. They also contain vitamins like B6 and folate, which play a role in immune cell production.

3. Legumes for Protein and Fiber

Legumes offer protein and complex carbs, making them an excellent choice for gut health and immune support. They're rich in fiber and resistant starch, which supports gut bacteria.

- Examples: Lentils, chickpeas, black beans, kidney beans.

- Benefits: Legumes provide a steady energy source, are high in fiber for gut health, and contain protein to support immune cell repair.

4. Berries for Antioxidant Power

While fruits are often higher in natural sugars, berries stand out because they are low on the glycemic index and packed with fiber and antioxidants.

- Examples: Blueberries, raspberries, strawberries, and blackberries.

- Benefits: Berries contain polyphenols, which have anti-inflammatory effects. They also support a balanced gut microbiome, indirectly boosting immune function.

Sample Recipes to Fuel Gut Repair and Cellular Vitality

Adding immune-boosting, gut-supportive carbs to your diet doesn't have to be complicated. Some simple, delicious recipes incorporate smart carbs to support cellular health.

Recipe 1: Fiber-Rich Breakfast Bowl

This fiber-packed breakfast bowl, with oats, berries, and chia seeds, supports gut health by providing a slow release of energy and essential nutrients.

Ingredients:

- 1/2 cup rolled oats

- 1 cup almond milk (or milk of choice)

- 1/4 cup mixed berries (blueberries, strawberries, or raspberries)

- 1 tbsp chia seeds

- 1 tsp honey (optional)

- 1/4 tsp cinnamon (for added antioxidants)

Instructions:

- In a bowl, combine oats and almond milk. Microwave for 1-2 minutes or heat on the stove until oats are soft.

- Top with berries, chia seeds, honey, and cinnamon.

- Stir well and enjoy a breakfast that fuels your gut and cells.

Recipe 2: Sweet Potato and Black Bean Power Bowl

This savory power bowl combines fiber-rich sweet potatoes with protein-packed black beans, supporting gut health and providing long-lasting energy.

Ingredients:

- 1 medium sweet potato, cubed

- 1/2 cup black beans, drained and rinsed

- 1/4 avocado, sliced

- 1 handful spinach

- 1 tbsp olive oil

- Salt and pepper, to taste

- Optional toppings: pumpkin seeds, a squeeze of lime, or a sprinkle of cilantro

Instructions:

- Preheat the oven to 400°F. Toss sweet potato cubes with olive oil, salt, and pepper, and roast for 25-30 minutes until tender.

- In a bowl, layer spinach, roasted sweet potato, black beans, and avocado slices.

- Top with optional garnishes like pumpkin seeds or cilantro for added nutrients.

Recipe 3: Gut-Friendly Lentil and Quinoa Salad

Packed with fiber and protein, this salad is an excellent lunch or dinner option that supports gut repair and strengthens immunity.

Ingredients:

- 1/2 cup cooked quinoa

- 1/2 cup cooked lentils

- 1/4 cucumber, diced

- 1/4 red bell pepper, diced

- 1 handful of arugula or spinach

- 1 tbsp olive oil

- Juice of 1/2 lemon

- Salt and pepper, to taste

Instructions:

- Combine quinoa, lentils, cucumber, bell pepper, and greens in a large bowl.

- Drizzle with olive oil and lemon juice. Season with salt and pepper.

- Toss and enjoy a refreshing, nutrient-dense salad that fuels your cells.

Daily Strategies to Support Protein Synthesis and Cell Repair

Carbohydrates and proteins support cellular repair, especially concerning immune cells and tissue regeneration. While carbohydrates provide the energy needed to fuel repair processes, protein provides the building blocks for cell regeneration and immune function.

Here's how to optimize this synergy in your daily life:

1. Pair Carbs with Protein

Eating carbs and protein together stabilizes blood sugar and supports protein synthesis. Protein synthesis is the process by which your body builds new proteins to replace worn-out or damaged ones.

- Example: Pair a handful of nuts (protein) with an apple (carb) as a snack, or combine chickpeas (protein) with brown rice (carb) in a salad.

2. Time Your Protein Intake

For optimal cell repair, especially after exercise or physical stress, consume a protein-rich meal within 30-60 minutes of activity. This timing maximizes protein synthesis and aids muscle repair, indirectly supporting cellular function and immunity.

- Example: A smoothie with protein powder and berries after a workout boosts recovery and supports immune health.

3. Include Essential Amino Acids in Each Meal

Your body relies on essential amino acids to build immune cells and repair tissues. While some amino acids can be synthesized by the body, essential amino acids must come from food. Including various protein sources ensures you get all the amino acids needed for optimal cellular repair.

Examples of Complete Proteins: Eggs, fish, lean meat, and quinoa. Combining incomplete proteins like rice and beans also provides a complete amino acid profile.

4. Incorporate B Vitamins for Energy Metabolism

B vitamins play a crucial role in energy production and cellular repair. They help convert carbs into usable energy and support synthesizing new cells, including immune cells.

- Sources of B Vitamins: Whole grains, leafy greens, eggs, and fortified cereals. Including these in your daily diet ensures your body has the resources for efficient cell repair and energy metabolism.

Final Thoughts on Gut Repair and Immune Strengthening

Strengthening your immune system and supporting cellular repair doesn't have to be complex. By incorporating intelligent carbs and choosing nutrient-dense foods, you provide your body with the tools it needs to thrive. These changes may seem small, but they have a cumulative impact on gut health, energy levels, and resilience against illness.

Incorporating complex, fiber-rich carbohydrates, pairing them with protein, and timing your meals to support protein synthesis will fuel your cells and help you build a lasting foundation of health.

A well-supported gut and a nourished immune system can help weather life's stressors with strength, focus, and vitality. Your cells are resilient and adaptive, and with the proper support, they will empower you to live a longer, happier life.

CHAPTER 11: Cellular-Boosting Supplements for Mitochondrial Health

Modern life can leave us feeling worn out and depleted as we contend with demanding schedules, environmental toxins, and, for many, inadequate nutrition. The cells in our bodies, especially our mitochondria—the powerhouses that produce cellular energy—require specific nutrients to function optimally.

Supplements can powerfully fill nutritional gaps and support cellular health, helping us regain energy, mental clarity, and resilience. In this chapter, we'll explore essential supplements that specifically support mitochondrial health, outline safe usage and potential side effects, and provide guidance on building a supplement routine to help you feel your best.

An Overview of Essential Vitamins and Supplements

Specific vitamins, minerals, and compounds stand out in terms of cellular health for their ability to support mitochondrial function, reduce oxidative stress, and promote energy production. Let's examine some of the most effective cellular-boosting supplements available today.

1. Coenzyme Q10 (CoQ10)

CoQ10 is an antioxidant naturally produced by the body and is crucial for energy production in our cells. It's concentrated in the mitochondria, where it helps generate ATP (adenosine triphosphate), the energy-carrying molecule that powers cellular functions. However, CoQ10 levels decline with age and can be depleted by certain medications, like statins.

- Benefits: Research shows that CoQ10 supplements can enhance energy levels, improve heart health, and reduce muscle fatigue. In older adults, CoQ10 can support cognitive health and may reduce symptoms of chronic fatigue.

- Usage: A typical dose is 100-300 mg daily, depending on your energy needs and overall health.

- Potential Side Effects: CoQ10 is generally safe, but in rare cases, it may cause digestive discomfort, nausea, or insomnia. It's best to start with a lower dose and take it with food to enhance absorption.

2. Magnesium

Magnesium is a mineral involved in over 300 enzymatic reactions, including those essential for mitochondrial energy production. It also supports muscle function, sleep quality, and stress management. Magnesium deficiency is expected due to modern diets and depleted soil; many people can benefit from supplementation.

- Benefits: Magnesium can improve sleep quality, reduce stress, and support energy production at the cellular level. It also helps with muscle relaxation and recovery, making it ideal for busy people.

- Usage: The recommended daily intake for adults is around 300-400 mg. Magnesium glycinate and magnesium citrate are often well-tolerated and highly absorbable.

- Potential Side Effects: High doses of magnesium, particularly from supplements, can cause digestive issues, including diarrhea. To avoid this, start with a lower dose and gradually increase as tolerated.

3. B-Vitamins (Especially B6, B12, and Folate)

B-vitamins are essential for cellular energy production, helping convert food into energy. They are essential in brain health, mood regulation, and mitochondrial function. B12 and folate are essential for people who experience fatigue, as deficiencies in these vitamins can lead to low energy levels and mental fog.

Benefits: Supplementing with B vitamins can improve mental clarity, energy, and mood. B12 and folate are especially beneficial for those on plant-based diets, as these nutrients are typically found in animal products.

- Usage: A daily B-complex supplement containing all essential B vitamins can be beneficial. B12 in the form of methylcobalamin is often recommended for its better bioavailability.

- Potential Side Effects: B vitamins are generally safe, as they're water-soluble, and excess amounts are excreted in urine. However, high doses of B6 may lead to nerve issues over time, so stick to recommended amounts.

4. Alpha-Lipoic Acid (ALA)

Alpha-lipoic acid is a powerful antioxidant that plays a role in mitochondrial energy production and helps regenerate other antioxidants, such as vitamins C and E. It's also known for its anti-inflammatory properties, which can help protect cells from oxidative stress.

- Benefits: ALA may improve energy levels, reduce inflammation, and support healthy blood sugar levels. It has been shown to support brain health and may improve memory and focus in older adults.

- Usage: A dose of 300-600 mg daily is commonly recommended. ALA is best taken on an empty stomach for optimal absorption.

- Potential Side Effects: Some people may experience mild digestive discomfort or a rash. High doses can affect thyroid function, so consult with a healthcare provider before using ALA if you have thyroid issues.

5. Acetyl-L-Carnitine (ALCAR)

Acetyl-L-carnitine is an amino acid derivative that supports energy production by transporting fatty acids into the mitochondria, which are burned for fuel. It's particularly beneficial for brain health, as it crosses the blood-brain barrier and may improve focus and memory.

- Benefits: Studies suggest that ALCAR can enhance mental clarity, reduce fatigue, and support cognitive function. It's often used by people who experience "brain fog" or struggle with concentration.

- Usage: A typical dose ranges from 500-1,500 mg daily, depending on your needs.

- Potential Side Effects: ALCAR is usually well-tolerated, but some may experience mild nausea or restlessness. Starting with a lower dose can help you gauge your body's response.

6. Vitamin D

Vitamin D is essential for immune function, bone health, and mood regulation. It also supports mitochondrial health, as studies show that cells need vitamin D to function optimally. Many people are deficient in vitamin D, particularly those in colder climates with limited sun exposure.

- Benefits: Vitamin D can improve energy, boost immunity, and support mental health. Adequate vitamin D levels are also associated with lower rates of chronic disease and better mitochondrial function.

- Usage: A typical dose is 1,000-2,000 IU per day, though some people may need higher amounts, especially if they have low baseline levels.

- Potential Side Effects: While vitamin D is safe at moderate doses, high levels can lead to toxicity. To ensure safe usage, check your vitamin D levels and supplement as needed.

Safe Usage and Potential Side Effects to Be Aware Of

As with any supplement, it's essential to consider the benefits and possible side effects. While supplements can be incredibly beneficial for cellular health, using them responsibly to avoid potential issues is crucial.

Here are some general tips to maximize safety:

- Start Slowly: When adding a new supplement, start with the lowest recommended dose to see how your body responds. This approach allows you to monitor any effects and adjust if needed.

- Stick to Quality Brands: Not all supplements are created equal. Choose reputable brands that have been third-party tested for purity and potency. Look for labels such as NSF Certified, USP Verified, or ConsumerLab.com approval, which indicate higher standards.

- Avoid Mega-Dosing: More is not always better when it comes to supplements. High doses of certain nutrients, like vitamin D or B6, can lead to toxicity over time. Follow recommended dosages and consult a healthcare provider if you're considering higher doses.

- Check for Interactions: Some supplements can interact with medications or other supplements. For instance, CoQ10 may interact with blood thinners, and high doses of magnesium can affect certain heart medications. If you take prescription medications, consult your doctor before adding new supplements.

- Cycle Your Supplements: Continuous use of some supplements may reduce their effectiveness over time. Consider taking breaks or rotating supplements to maintain their benefits. For instance, you might take Alpha-Lipoic Acid for three months, then pause for a month before resuming.

Building a Supplement Routine for Daily Energy and Health

Creating a supplement routine that works for you doesn't have to be complicated. Here's a sample routine that incorporates some of the top mitochondrial-supporting supplements mentioned above:

Morning

- Vitamin D (1,000-2,000 IU): Start your day by taking vitamin D, as it's best absorbed with a meal containing healthy fats.

- B-Complex Vitamin: Take a high-quality B-complex vitamin to kickstart energy production and support brain function.

- Alpha-Lipoic Acid (300 mg): Take on an empty stomach to enhance absorption and support mitochondrial energy production.

Afternoon

- Acetyl-L-Carnitine (500-1,000 mg): A mid-day dose of ALCAR can help maintain mental clarity and combat afternoon fatigue.

- Magnesium (200-300 mg): Magnesium can help manage stress, support muscle function, and promote sustained energy throughout the day.

Evening

- Coenzyme Q10 (100 mg): Taking CoQ10 with your evening meal helps improve absorption and supports cellular energy production overnight.

- Herbal Tea: Consider winding down with a cup of dandelion tea, which supports liver function and gentle detoxification.

Adjusting Your Routine Based on Your Needs

This routine is simply a starting point. You can adjust the timing and combination of supplements depending on your unique health needs, lifestyle, and goals. For example, if you struggle with sleep, taking magnesium in the evening might be more beneficial for relaxation. Or, if your primary concern is mental clarity, you might prioritize acetyl-L-carnitine and B vitamins.

Tracking Your Progress

One of the best ways to see if a supplement routine is effective is by monitoring your feelings. Keep a journal or make mental notes about changes in energy, focus, mood, and physical health. Notice if you feel less fatigued, more focused, or more resilient to stress. These improvements are signs that your cells are benefiting from the support.

Empowering Your Cells for a Life of Vitality

Supplements aren't magic pills but can significantly support mitochondrial health, energy production, and overall cellular function. By choosing high-quality supplements and using them mindfully, you're empowering your cells to perform at their best, translating into more energy, focus, and resilience in your daily life.

Remember, cellular health is a long-term investment. With each step you take—from eating nutritious foods to incorporating targeted supplements—you're building a foundation of health that will support you for years to come. Embrace this journey, and enjoy the renewed vitality of nurturing your body at the cellular level.

CHAPTER 12: Empowering Your Metabolism – The 30-Day Cellular Health Plan

In our fast-paced world, many people feel trapped in fatigue, brain fog, and low energy cycles. Despite trying various diets, exercise routines, and supplements, they're left frustrated by fleeting results and discouraged by complex health advice that seems unrealistic.

This chapter is designed with you in mind. It offers a structured, 30-day plan to support cellular health and metabolic function. Think of this as a "reset" to help you jumpstart your energy and establish sustainable habits that will empower your metabolism and keep your cells thriving.

This step-by-step plan is realistic, flexible, and designed to fit into your daily life. By following it, you'll build a solid foundation of cellular health, improve energy levels, and boost overall vitality. Here's how you can experience a transformative journey over the next 30 days.

A Step-by-Step Plan to Jumpstart Your Cellular Renewal

In this 30-day plan, each week is dedicated to specific goals that build upon each other, creating a comprehensive approach to cellular health. By focusing on different aspects of cellular wellness—from nutrition to movement, stress management to hydration—you'll address the key factors that impact metabolism, cellular function, and energy levels.

Week 1: Nutrition Foundation for Cellular Health

In the first week, we'll focus on establishing a nutrition foundation that supports cellular health. Choosing foods rich in essential nutrients will nourish your cells and empower your body to perform optimally.

Day 1-3: Eliminate Processed Foods

Processed foods contain additives and preservatives that can impair cellular function. Focus on whole foods like vegetables, fruits, lean proteins, and whole grains. For example, try replacing sugary snacks with fresh fruit or swapping out white bread for whole-grain options. This will help your cells receive the nutrients they need without added toxins.

Day 4-7: Add Nutrient-Rich Foods

Begin incorporating foods that directly support cellular health, such as leafy greens (rich in chlorophyll), nuts (packed with healthy fats), and berries (high in antioxidants). These foods provide cells with vital nutrients that support energy production and reduce oxidative stress.

- Weekly Tip: Create a "cellular health plate" with each meal by filling half of your plate with colorful vegetables, a quarter with lean protein, and the remaining quarter with whole grains. This balanced approach ensures you support your metabolism and cellular function with every meal.

Week 2: Movement and Circulation

In the second week, we'll focus on integrating movement into your daily routine. Movement increases circulation, which delivers oxygen and nutrients to cells, boosts metabolism, and supports detoxification. These benefits are essential for cellular health and overall energy levels.

Day 8-10: Start with Light Exercise

If you're inactive, begin with light exercises such as walking, stretching, or yoga. Aim for 20–30 minutes each day. For example, a brisk walk after lunch or gentle yoga in the morning can help wake up your metabolism and promote cellular energy.

Day 11-14: Add Strength Training

Strength training supports muscle health and boosts metabolism by increasing muscle mass, which burns more calories at rest. Try adding two 20-minute sessions of bodyweight exercises, such as squats, lunges, or push-ups. Strength training enhances metabolic function and supports bone health and mental clarity.

Weekly Tip: Schedule exercise as an essential part of your day. Consistency is more important than duration, even if you can only fit in 10–15 minutes. Movement fuels cellular health, and the benefits will compound over time.

Week 3: Hydration and Detoxification

Hydration and detoxification are critical for cellular health. Proper hydration allows cells to efficiently carry out metabolic functions, while detoxification helps remove toxins that can impair cellular function. This week, we will focus on practical hydration and detox strategies that can be easily incorporated into daily life.

Day 15-17: Increase Water Intake

Drinking water supports cellular processes and helps flush out toxins. Aim for at least 8–10 glasses daily, and add a slice of lemon for extra antioxidants. For example, start your day with a glass of water to rehydrate after sleep and sip throughout the day to maintain energy.

Day 18-21: Add Detoxifying Foods

Include foods naturally supporting detoxification, such as garlic, ginger, and green tea. Garlic contains sulfur compounds that support liver function, while ginger aids digestion and reduces inflammation. Green tea is rich in antioxidants, which help neutralize toxins and support cellular resilience.

- Weekly Tip: If plain water feels monotonous, try infusing it with fresh herbs like mint, basil, or cucumber for added flavor and detox benefits. Staying hydrated will support digestion, energy, and mental clarity, all essential for cellular health.

Week 4: Stress Management and Restorative Practices

Stress management and sleep are often overlooked in cellular health, but they play crucial roles. Chronic stress and poor sleep disrupt cellular processes and contribute to fatigue and low energy. This week, we will focus on incorporating practices that reduce stress and improve rest.

Day 22-25: Begin a Daily Mindfulness Practice

Mindfulness practices such as meditation or deep breathing reduce stress hormones like cortisol, which can impair cellular function over time. Set aside 5–10 minutes each morning to practice mindfulness. For example, try deep breathing or guided meditation to start your day with a calm mind.

Day 26-28: Establish a Restful Night Routine

Prioritize sleep by creating a relaxing bedtime routine. Limit screen time before bed, and try reading or practicing gentle stretches instead. Aim for 7–8 hours of quality sleep each night, as this is when cellular repair processes are most active.

- Weekly Tip: Even minor adjustments to your stress management and sleep routines can make a difference. Quality sleep and stress reduction allow your cells to repair, helping you wake up with more energy and clarity.

Daily Practices to Boost Energy, Mood, and Vitality

By following these structured weekly goals, you'll be supporting your cells on multiple levels. The following daily practices are designed to maintain the momentum you've built through each plan phase.

- Morning Hydration Ritual: Start each day with a glass of water and a splash of lemon to support hydration and kickstart detoxification.

- Balanced Breakfast for Sustained Energy: Eat a nutrient-dense breakfast, such as oatmeal topped with berries and a handful of nuts. This combination of fiber, healthy fats, and antioxidants supports stable blood sugar levels, promoting steady energy and focus throughout the morning.

- Midday Movement: Take a short walk or stretch break to keep your circulation active and support cellular oxygen delivery. Even a 10-minute break helps counteract the effects of prolonged sitting.

- Mindfulness Breaks: Incorporate two or three short mindfulness sessions daily, especially if stress creeps in. Simple breathing exercises or brief meditation sessions can reset your focus, reduce stress, and improve your mood.

- Evening Wind-Down: As you wrap up each day, focus on activities that relax and restore you, such as reading, journaling, or practicing gratitude. A calm evening supports more profound, restorative sleep, allowing your cells to repair and rejuvenate.

Tracking Progress and Celebrating Your Health Journey

Tracking your changes as you progress through the 30-day plan can help you stay motivated and see the impact of your efforts. Here's a simple method for tracking your progress and celebrating each step along the way.

1. Energy Journal

At the start of your journey, write down how you currently feel—energy levels, mood, mental clarity, and overall well-being. Each day, take a moment to jot down any noticeable changes, no matter how small. You may be surprised by how these incremental shifts add up to a significant improvement in your health and vitality.

2. Weekly Reflection

At the end of each week, reflect on the habits you've established and the changes you've noticed. Use this time to celebrate your progress and set intentions for the following week. Reflecting helps reinforce your commitment and allows you to adjust your goals to better fit your needs.

3. Celebrate Small Wins

It's easy to overlook the small wins, but each positive change represents progress in your health journey. Acknowledge these wins, whether it's an increase in energy, improved sleep, or just feeling better overall. Reward yourself meaningfully, like taking time for a favorite activity or a nourishing meal.

4. Evaluate and Adjust

After completing the 30 days, take a moment to evaluate the practices that had the most positive impact on your life. Which habits felt sustainable? Which areas need more focus? Use these reflections to build a lifestyle supporting your cellular health beyond the 30-day plan.

Embrace Your Cellular Health Journey

The journey to cellular health isn't a sprint; it's a lifelong commitment to treating your body with the care it deserves. As you've seen through this plan, health isn't just about temporary solutions or drastic overhauls—it's about small, sustainable habits that nourish and support you daily.

Each step is a piece of the larger picture, contributing to your energy, resilience, and overall vitality. By nurturing your cells, you're setting a foundation that empowers you to live a life full of purpose and joy.

Whether you feel the immediate benefits or slowly build a stronger, healthier foundation, know that every effort you put in is worth it. As your cells thrive, so will you. Embrace the journey, celebrate your progress, and remember that health and vitality are within reach—one day, one habit at a time.

Chapter 13: Thriving in a Modern World – Sustaining Cellular Health

As you conclude your journey through cellular health, you must recognize that maintaining vibrant health is an ongoing process, especially in a world of daily stressors that impact our cells.

While you've learned how to detoxify, nourish, and energize your cells, life's demands, environmental challenges, and even social influences can create obstacles.

This chapter will guide you in developing strategies to keep your cells thriving amid modern stressors. We'll explore sustainable lifestyle habits for long-term health and provide you with resources and tools for continued success.

By understanding how to address these challenges, you'll be equipped to create a life where cellular health isn't a temporary goal but a permanent foundation for vitality and longevity.

Addressing Modern Stressors That Impact Cellular Well-Being

Our bodies and cells constantly adapt to the conditions around us, but today's world presents unique challenges our ancestors didn't face. To sustain cellular health, it's essential to recognize these modern stressors and understand how to mitigate their effects.

1. Environmental Toxins

From pollution in the air to chemicals in our food and water, environmental toxins are among the most prevalent challenges to cellular health today. These toxins accumulate in our cells, impairing mitochondrial function and leading to oxidative stress—two factors that can accelerate aging and weaken overall health.

Practical Tips for Reducing Toxin Exposure:

- Filter Your Water: A high-quality water filter can help remove contaminants like heavy metals, pesticides, and chlorine from tap water. Filtering your water protects your cells and improves hydration by eliminating compounds that could otherwise hinder cellular absorption.

- Choose Organic Produce: Where possible, opt for organic fruits and vegetables to reduce exposure to pesticides and herbicides. The Environmental Working Group's (EWG) "Dirty Dozen" list highlights the produce items with the highest pesticide levels, making prioritizing organic options for the most affected items easier.

- Detox Your Living Space: Indoor air can be up to five times more polluted than outdoor air, so investing in an air purifier and adding indoor plants (such as snake plants, peace lilies, or spider plants) can help remove toxins from the air you breathe daily.

2. Digital Overload and Electromagnetic Fields (EMFs)

The convenience of technology is invaluable, yet the constant exposure to screens, blue light, and EMFs from devices has been shown to contribute to cellular stress. Digital overload affects both mental and physical health, leading to sleep disturbances, mental fatigue, and even cell damage over time.

Ways to Protect Yourself from Digital Overload:

- Establish Screen-Free Times: Designate specific times of the day to unplug. For example, aim to turn off all screens at least one hour before bedtime to support healthy melatonin levels, which regulate sleep and play a role in cellular repair.

- Use Blue Light Filters: Many devices now have built-in blue light filters that reduce eye strain. Additionally, consider using blue light-blocking glasses, primarily if you work on a computer for extended periods.

- Limit EMF Exposure: While avoiding EMFs completely is impossible, you can reduce exposure by keeping electronic devices away from your bed at night, using speakerphone or wired headsets instead of holding your phone to your ear, and avoiding carrying your phone directly on your body.

3. Chronic Stress and Cortisol Overload

Stress is a normal part of life, but it can create a cascade of cellular issues when it becomes chronic. High cortisol levels from chronic stress contribute to inflammation, disrupt sleep patterns, and weaken immune function. Over time, elevated cortisol can impair cellular repair processes and even alter gene expression.

Strategies to Manage and Reduce Stress:

- Practice Mindfulness or Meditation: Research shows that mindfulness meditation reduces cortisol levels and improves resilience to stress. Even five minutes a day can create a noticeable difference. Apps like Headspace and Calm provide guided meditations, making starting this practice easy and accessible.

- Engage in Physical Activity: Exercise is a powerful stress reducer. Activities like yoga, walking, or swimming alleviate stress and increase blood flow, delivering more oxygen to your cells and supporting cellular health.

- Set Boundaries: Modern work culture often blurs the lines between work and personal life. Setting clear boundaries—such as no work emails after a particular time or scheduling regular breaks—can prevent burnout and protect your mental and cellular health.

Creating a Sustainable Lifestyle for Long-Term Health

Consistency is critical to cellular health, but creating a lifestyle that supports long-term wellness doesn't have to be complicated or restrictive. By building habits that become part of your routine, you can nurture your cells daily without feeling overwhelmed or frustrated.

1. Adopt a Nutrient-Dense Diet for Daily Cellular Support

Choosing whole, nutrient-dense foods gives your cells the vitamins, minerals, and antioxidants they need to function optimally. Aim to make your meals a source of cellular support rather than stress.

Examples of Nutrient-Rich Foods for Cellular Health:

- Leafy Greens: Spinach, kale, and arugula are rich in vitamins A, C, and K, which support cellular repair and antioxidant protection.

- Healthy Fats: Avocados, olive oil, and nuts are high in monounsaturated fats, which nourish cell membranes and enhance cellular resilience.

- Colorful Fruits and Vegetables: Berries, sweet potatoes, and bell peppers contain antioxidants that protect against oxidative stress.

2. Make Movement a Daily Priority

Exercise is one of the most effective ways to enhance cellular health. It increases circulation, reduces inflammation, and boosts mitochondrial function. Rather than treating exercise as a chore, view it as an essential tool for keeping your cells energized and healthy.

Sustainable Exercise Tips:

- Find What You Enjoy: Choose activities that you look forward to. Whether dancing, hiking, or practicing yoga, enjoying your movement routine increases the likelihood of consistency.

- Incorporate Movement Breaks: If you work at a desk, take short breaks every hour to stretch, walk around, or do a few squats. These small moments of activity reduce the strain of prolonged sitting, which has been linked to cellular aging.

- Practice Active Recovery: Gentle activities like stretching, walking, and foam rolling can help prevent injury and ensure your body remains limber and ready for more intense exercise sessions.

3. Prioritize Rest and Recovery

Sleep is when most cellular repair occurs, and without adequate rest, cells struggle to regenerate and function effectively. Establishing a sleep routine can be transformative, providing the foundation your cells need to recover from daily stressors.

Ways to Improve Sleep for Better Cellular Health:

- Create a Relaxing Bedtime Routine: Start winding down at least an hour before bed. Dim the lights, avoid screens, and do calming activities like reading or meditating.

- Keep a Consistent Schedule: Going to bed and waking up simultaneously every day reinforces your body's circadian rhythm, improving sleep quality over time.

- Optimize Your Sleep Environment: A calm, dark, quiet bedroom promotes restful sleep. To reduce disruptions, use blackout curtains, a white noise machine, or an eye mask.

Tools and Resources for Continued Cellular Health Success

As you move forward, maintaining cellular health will become a natural part of your life. To support you on this journey, here are some additional tools, resources, and practices to help you continue thriving.

1. Tracking Your Progress

Documenting changes in your energy levels, mood, and health can be motivating and insightful. Consider keeping a health journal or using a wellness app to track your progress and recognize patterns.

Examples of Tools for Health Tracking:

- Apps like MyFitnessPal or Cronometer: These can help you track nutrient intake and ensure you're getting the vitamins and minerals your cells need.

- Sleep Tracking Apps: Apps like Sleep Cycle or Oura Ring can provide insights into sleep quality, helping you identify habits that enhance your rest and cellular recovery.

- Heart Rate Variability (HRV) Monitors: HRV indicates stress and resilience. Higher HRV is associated with better cellular health and stress management. Fitness devices like Fitbit, WHOOP, or Garmin offer HRV tracking.

2. Building a Support System

Maintaining cellular health can be more enjoyable and sustainable when shared with others. Connecting with friends, family, or online communities sharing similar health goals can provide accountability and encouragement.

Ways to Find Support:

- Join Online Forums or Groups: Platforms like Reddit and Facebook host communities focused on cellular health, nutrition, and longevity where you can share experiences and ask questions.

- Attend Wellness Classes or Workshops: Many local health and wellness centers offer classes or workshops on topics such as cellular nutrition, stress management, and detoxification.

- Partner Up: Having a health buddy can make lifestyle changes fun and less daunting. Whether it's a friend, family member, or coworker, partnering up can help you stay motivated.

3. Staying Informed and Inspired

Cellular health science is continually evolving, and staying updated on the latest research and practices can empower you to make informed decisions that benefit your health.

Recommended Resources for Ongoing Learning:

- Podcasts: Shows like The Model Health Show, The Ultimate Health Podcast, and FoundMyFitness explore the science of health and longevity.

- Books and Articles: Look for reputable sources of information on cellular health, like scientific journals or publications by trusted nutrition and integrative medicine experts.

- Continuing Education: Workshops, online courses, and certifications can expand your knowledge. Platforms like Coursera, Udemy, and the Institute for Integrative Nutrition offer holistic health and wellness classes.

Embracing Cellular Health for Life

Congratulations on reaching this point in your journey. By understanding the foundations of cellular health, you've equipped yourself with tools for a life filled with energy, resilience, and longevity. Remember, thriving in a modern world isn't about adhering to perfection—it's about making intentional choices that support your cells day after day.

Your commitment to cellular health is one of the most impactful decisions you can make for your future. As you continue, let these practices become part of who you are, sustaining you through life's ups and downs. Embrace each step, knowing that every small action brings you closer to a life of vitality and well-being. Here's to thriving every single day.

CONCLUSION: Embracing the Power of Cellular Health for a Life of Vitality and Joy

As you reach the end of The Power of Cellular Health: Secrets to a Longer, Happier Life, I hope you feel inspired and empowered to take charge of your health at the cellular level.

By now, you've learned that vitality doesn't come from quick fixes or temporary measures—it starts from within, from the most minor units that make up our bodies. By nurturing our cells, we're creating a foundation of health that sustains energy, focus, and joy.

The journey you've embarked upon isn't just about adding years to your life; it's about enhancing the quality of those years. Cellular health gives us the remarkable opportunity to age gracefully, to enjoy each moment, and to live with resilience and strength.

For many, the journey began with struggles: the frustration of unexplained fatigue, the mental fog that makes even the simplest tasks feel insurmountable, or the aches and pains we're told are just a part of "getting older." But these are not inevitable. As you've discovered in these pages, many of these challenges are rooted in how well our cells function, and we have the power to support them.

Honoring Your Body's Potential

Our bodies are remarkably resilient and capable of change. Our cells work daily to repair, renew, and protect us. Even as we age, this process continues. Our cells can do incredible things with the right support—from proper nutrition to stress management, from mindful movement to restorative sleep.

Imagine each cell as a dedicated worker, giving you the energy to play with your kids or grandkids, the focus to tackle a demanding project, or the strength to stay active in the things you love. These possibilities are within reach, regardless of where you start today.

I hope this book has shown you there is always potential for improvement and growth. Whether you've started making small changes or overhauling your habits, every step you take contributes to your long-term well-being. Cellular health isn't about perfection; it's about progress. Each new practice you implement, each nourishing meal you choose, and each mindful moment you spend on self-care moves you closer to the vibrant life you envision.

A Lifelong Commitment to Wellness

Adopting a cellular health approach means committing to yourself and your well-being most fundamentally. This journey doesn't end with finishing this book; it's just beginning.

Maintaining cellular health is a lifelong process that evolves as you do. Life may present challenges—busy seasons, periods of stress, or unexpected health issues—but remember that the tools and strategies you've learned here are designed to adapt with you.

As you continue your journey, be kind to yourself. If there are times when you fall back into old habits, that's okay. What's important is knowing that you have a roadmap to return to, centered around nourishing and supporting your body at its foundation.

Cellular health offers flexibility, allowing you to make adjustments as needed. Ultimately, the goal isn't rigid adherence to any single approach but the freedom to make choices that support your health and happiness.

Celebrating the Small Wins

As you apply these principles, remember to celebrate each milestone, no matter how small it may seem. Perhaps you've noticed more energy during the day, clearer thinking, or better sleep. These are significant achievements, signs that your cells are responding to the care you give them.

It's easy to overlook these improvements in our fast-paced world, but they're worth acknowledging. Small, positive changes add up over time, creating a solid foundation of health that can support you for years to come.

Each success, each slight improvement, brings you closer to your ideal state of health and vitality. Let these moments remind you of your impact on your life. Cellular health isn't a destination; it's a continuous journey that enables you to feel and live better with each passing day.

As you move forward, keep exploring and stay curious. Cellular health science is continuously evolving, with new research shedding light on even more ways to optimize our well-being. You've taken the essential first steps by building a foundation of cellular health knowledge and practices. Now, you can confidently build upon this foundation, integrating new insights as they come to light.

Remember, this book is here as a resource, something you can return to whenever you need guidance or encouragement. Whether revisiting a favorite chapter on mitochondrial health or re-reading tips on reducing inflammation, this guide supports you at every stage.

And as you progress, your knowledge and intuition about your body will only grow stronger. You'll come to recognize what your body needs, how to nourish it, and how to listen to the subtle signals that guide you toward health.

Final Words of Encouragement

The journey to cellular health is one of your most meaningful commitments. Every decision to prioritize your cells—whether by choosing nutritious foods, taking time to rest, or managing stress—is a step toward living a life of vitality and purpose. You have the power to shape your health, protect and energize your body, and live a life that not only spans years but is filled with quality, joy, and fulfillment.

Imagine the freedom of waking up each day feeling energized and capable, the satisfaction of knowing you're investing in your future, and the peace of mind that comes from knowing you're doing everything you can to support your health. Cellular health gives you these gifts, empowering you to live fully at every age.

Share Your Journey with Others

This book has inspired and empowered you to embrace cellular health in your own life. If you've found value in these pages, I'd like your help. By leaving a review of The Power of Cellular Health on Amazon, you're doing more than just sharing your thoughts—you're helping others find this book and join the journey toward a healthier, more vibrant life.

Reviews are incredibly important for helping books reach a wider audience, and your honest feedback can make a difference.

Your experience and insights can help guide others struggling with the same pain points—fatigue, stress, aging concerns, or simply the desire for a more energetic, fulfilling life. By sharing what you've learned, you're contributing to a community of people working toward their best selves.

If this book has helped you, even in small ways, please leave a review. Your words may encourage someone else to begin their journey to cellular health. Together, we can create a ripple effect, spreading health, vitality, and happiness one cell at a time.

Thank you for taking this journey with me and for being part of the movement toward a healthier, more joyful world. Here's to your cellular health, vitality, and the extraordinary life ahead.

9 798345 425381